ANABOLIC STEROIDS

ANABOLIC STEROIDS AND OTHER PERFORMANCE- ENHANCING DRUGS

PAT LENEHAN

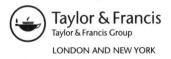

Taylor & Francis
Taylor & Francis Group

LONDON AND NEW YORK

First published 2003 by Taylor & Francis
11 New Fetter Lane, London EC4P 4EE

Simultaneously published in the USA and Canada
by Taylor & Francis Inc,
29 West 35th Street, New York, NY 10001

Taylor & Francis is an imprint of the Taylor & Francis Group

© 2003 Taylor & Francis

Typeset in 11/12pt Garamond 3
by Graphicraft Limited, Hong Kong
Printed and bound in Great Britain by Biddles Ltd, Guildford and King's Lynn

Every effort has been made to ensure that the advice and information in this book is
true and accurate at the time of going to press. However, neither the publisher nor the
authors can accept any legal responsibility or liability for any errors or omissions that
may be made. In the case of drug administration, any medical procedure or the use
of technical equipment mentioned within this book, you are strongly advised to consult
the manufacturer's guidelines.

British Library Cataloguing in Publication Data
A catalogue record for this book is available from the British Library

Library of Congress Cataloging in Publication Data
A catalogue entry has been requested

ISBN 0-415-28029-X (hbk)
ISBN 0-415-28030-3 (pbk)

To

Mum, Di and Marian

for everything

I have been very fortunate in meeting a number of people who have been incredibly supportive of my professional endeavours over the years; some have become very good friends. The list is very long but in particular I would like to thank Jim, Rod, Mark, Pirkko, Pat, Bruce, Clive, Steve, Iain, Brendan, Howard, Stuart and Ian.

Contents

CHAPTER 1

Introduction

This book is designed to provide information about the use of anabolic steroids and some of the other drugs that are used in conjunction with them. I have tried to keep the book accessible to all readers so I have attempted to keep the amount of technical jargon to a minimum but on occasions it has proven necessary to include some medical, chemical or biological terminology. My own interest in performance-enhancing drugs has developed over the past fifteen years, less from their use in sport than in their non-competitive use. This is discussed in more detail later.

The book has four parts:

1 An overview of the social history of anabolic steroids including their development, prevalence and implications for society.
2 The medical side-effects of the use of anabolic steroids, both physical and psychological.
3 It is impossible to discuss the issue of anabolic steroids without making reference to sport. Traditionally, the use of these drugs has been considered to be almost exclusively the domain of sportsmen. It also affords the opportunity of using the banned drug list of the International Olympic Committee as a framework to discuss other performance-enhancing drugs.
4 The final section looks at how anabolic steroids are used, other performance-enhancing drugs and supplements, a discussion of the problems associated with counterfeit drugs and drug profiles of some of the more commonly used drugs.

1.1 *What are anabolic steroids?*

The effects of anabolic steroids mimic those of testosterone. Naturally synthesized hormones, such as testosterone, are types of lipids. They have a four-ring carbon skeleton and are synthesized in the adrenal cortex, ovaries or testes. Production of testosterone takes place in the male testes and the female ovaries; it is present in the male at significantly higher levels than in females, two of the main effects being androgenic and anabolic.

> **Androgenic** changes involve secondary sexual characteristics in the male (e.g. facial hair and deepening of the voice).
> **Anabolic** changes include the growth and development of many body tissues, perhaps most obviously muscles.

The production of testosterone is itself stimulated by another hormone, luteinizing hormone, produced in the pituitary. As well as controlling the growth, development and function of the male sex organs, testosterone and the other hormones present are responsible for the 'masculinizing' or 'virilizing' effects of male puberty. When males reach the end of puberty, the amount of testosterone rises suddenly and stays at a high level for four to six months before returning to normal. During this time, the growth plates in the long bones of the arms and legs close, the voice deepens, facial hair begins to grow and the male sex organs grow in size. It is this surge in testosterone that completes the sexual maturation of males.

At one time, researchers thought that anabolic and androgenic steroids were different. It was thought that chemists could create new versions of steroids to build up muscle tissue without causing masculine side-effects. However, they discovered that anabolic and androgenic effects were both caused by the same drug action on different tissue types. Thus, any anabolic steroid that builds up muscle tissue also causes masculinizing side-effects. Because of the possible impact on women and children prescribed anabolic steroids therapeutically, synthetic steroids are manufactured to enhance their anabolic but diminish their androgenic properties, although they cannot be entirely suppressed. Therefore, it is more correct to call this group of drugs anabolic-androgenic steroids (AAS); however, for the purposes of this book I continue to call them anabolic steroids (AS).

1.2 *Why a book about anabolic steroids?*

Anabolic steroids have been used in sport since the 1950s but their use has long ceased to be solely a sporting problem. For instance, it was estimated in

1993 that 83,000 11–18-year-old Canadians had taken them during that year (Melia, 1994). Drug use among those involved in health and fitness is perceived to be a Europe-wide public health issue (Council of Europe, 1998, 2001), although precise data on the prevalence of their use are lacking. Studies in Britain estimate that up to 50% of gym users may have taken them at some time (Korkia and Stimson, 1993; Lenehan *et al.*, 1996). A survey of 1000 school children in Sefton in the north-west of England showed that AS were the third most commonly offered drug behind cannabis and amphetamines (Clarke, 1999) and had been offered to 6.4% of boys and 1.3% of girls, suggesting that the potential for AS use has gone beyond the gym setting.

The majority of AS users inject the drug (Korkia and Stimson, 1993; Lenehan *et al.*, 1996; Dawson, 2001) and needle-exchange schemes have been known to provide AS injectors with advice and free sterile injecting equipment. In 1995, they were the second most commonly injected drug encountered by services in the Liverpool area (Lenehan *et al.*, 1996). The Drug Misuse Database for Merseyside and North Cheshire confirms that the trend for more AS users attending needle exchanges continues and that in 2001, for the first time, more AS users attended these services than opiate users (J. McVeigh, personal communication). In the North-East, 60% of people accessing needle-exchange services were AS injectors (Dawson, 2001).

Anabolic steroid use may be implicated in increased mortality and morbidity (Parssinen *et al.*, 2000). Besides the use of black market drugs of unknown quality and content (Perry, 1995), concurrent use of additional illicit drugs is also common among AS users. The use of drugs in conjunction with anabolic steroids has also been linked to increased aggression and violence. Black market drugs carry an additional and sometimes an extreme health risk (Perry and Hughes, 1992).

It is clear that the prevalence of AS use could have a significant impact on society. Many of the issues relating to this issue remain unaddressed. The increasing prevalence of AS use among adolescents presents a major cause for concern. There appears to be inadequate provision of services for AS users in the UK; previous studies have noted how inaccessible this group of drug users can be to health professionals (Best and Henderson, 1995; McVeigh and Lenehan, 1995; Lenehan *et al.*, 1996). This may present particular problems in terms of availability of clean injecting equipment, advice, general medical help, and treatments for AS withdrawal. There have already been reports of HIV being contracted as a result of AS users sharing injecting equipment (Sklarek *et al.*, 1984; Scott and Scott, 1989; Henrion *et al.*, 1992), and the incidence of this means of contracting infections may be underestimated.

Even though there is evidence that AS use is widespread in the UK, there are few reliable sources of information for users and health professionals alike. I hope that this book will go some way to redress this situation.

CHAPTER 2

Social history of anabolic steroids

Anabolic steroids (AS) have been used for a variety of therapeutic and non-therapeutic purposes. AS are derivatives of the male sex hormone, testosterone. In the mid-1930s two research groups, Ruzicka and Wettstein and Butenandt and Hanisch, isolated androstenedione and converted it to what is now known as testosterone. Following this research the anabolic properties of testosterone were documented (Kochakian, 1935, 1975; Kochakian and Murlin, 1935). Since these discoveries, various research groups have made modifications to the basic structure of testosterone and produced a range of closely related compounds that are marketed as anabolic steroids. The purpose of the majority of these modifications has been to dissociate the androgenic (masculinizing) properties from the anabolic properties, although this has not yet been successfully achieved (Kochakian, 1993a).

2.1 Early discoveries of the anabolic and androgenic properties of testosterone

Primitive medicine holds an early clue about the medical applications of testosterone. The practice of treating an organ with itself, also known as similia similibus, or organotherapy, was frequently applied by the ancient Greeks, and later by the Romans, to treat a wide variety of complaints. Human or animal tissues would be used to treat various complaints; for example, the eating of brain tissue was recommended to improve a low intellect (Newerla, 1943; Hoberman and Yesalis, 1995). The centuries-old practice of castration provided evidence that the testes were involved in the development of secondary male sex characteristics (Hoskins, 1941). This knowledge led to the belief that the consumption of testicular tissue could be used to treat an array of complaints, specifically including impotence (Taylor, 1991). These practices were also applied to the improvement of sporting performance. Athletes in ancient Greece would eat lambs' testes in an attempt to increase their strength and muscle size. Further medical and scientific discoveries served to reduce the frequency with which these practices were applied, but interest in the effects of testicular extracts and testes transplantation has continued. The use of animal experimentation to provide a model of testicular function and hormonal regulation is still applied today, and experiments involving human subjects are often conducted.

Some of the earliest experiments to investigate the function of the testes were conducted by Berthold in the mid-nineteenth century. He conducted experiments with roosters and showed that transplantation of testes into castrated roosters (capons) led to regression of the changes that occurred as a result of castration, namely the regrowth of comb and wattles and changes in behaviour. Berthold concluded that a secretion from the transplanted testis was responsible for these changes. Berthold's experiments were repeated by different scientists with variable success. Eventually, Berthold's conclusions were verified, as a result of work by McGee (1927) and Gallagher and Koch (1934). Both of these groups conducted modified versions of the Berthold experiment, in which they used an alcohol extract of bull testicle to stimulate the regrowth of the combs of castrated roosters. Following research that proved extracts from men's urine had a similar stimulatory effect upon regrowth of the comb of castrated roosters (Ruzicka *et al.*, 1934), it became accepted that the testes produced an active extract responsible for the development and maintenance of male characteristics (Kochakian, 1993b).

2.2 *Effects of testicular extract (testosterone) and related substances upon humans*

A number of experiments were carried out in the nineteenth century by Brown-Sequard, a French physiologist, in which he injected the aqueous extracts from animal testes into himself as well as into a range of animals. In 1889 Brown-Sequard reported his observations, declaring that he had reversed his own decline into old age. Although Brown-Sequard's discoveries were not accepted because of the lack of experimental controls, his idea that the testes release physiologically active substances proved to be true (Kochakian, 1993a). His self-experimentation provided the basis for further studies into the effects of ingestion of testicular extracts, and ultimately the effects of testosterone, upon people.

Surgeons developed the technique of transplanting human and animal (e.g. monkeys) testes into patients whose testes were damaged or dysfunctional. Claims were made that these operations had relieved pain and discomfort and promoted bodily well-being in hundreds of patients. People began to seek treatment for all manner of disorders: senility, asthma, epilepsy, diabetes, impotence, tuberculosis, paranoia, gangrene and more (Hoberman and Yesalis, 1995). However, this method of treatment was not accepted by the scientific community, who did not believe many of the claims made. An international committee that was appointed to investigate these claims concluded that claims of rejuvenation as a result of testicular transplantation were unfounded (Parkes, 1985). Subsequent to the research outlined above, testosterone has been isolated and its structure discovered.

2.3 Early uses of testosterone and its derivatives

There are rumours that German soldiers were administered anabolic steroids during the Second World War, the aim being to increase their aggression and stamina (Yesalis *et al.*, 1993a). These rumours have often been reported (Verroken, 1996) but are, as yet, unproven. Hitler was also believed to have been treated by his physician with injections of testosterone (Taylor, 1991). A more ethical application of anabolic steroid treatment was also applied at the end of the Second World War, whereby these drugs were used to treat the malnourished victims of the Nazi concentration camps (George, 1996a).

Other early uses were found for testosterone derivatives in the treatment of men and women with abnormal hormone production. The mode of action of these treatments works on almost identical principles to the primitive transplantation of testicular tissue; exogenous testosterone circulates around the body to fulfil the roles of endogenous testosterone. The first documented case of testosterone being used to treat a patient was by Hamilton (1937). This physician administered a total of 550 mg of testosterone acetate, given via 14 injections with three injections per week, to a 27-year-old male patient who was suffering from sexual underdevelopment (hypogonadism). Hamilton's experiment proved to be successful, the patient experienced penile erections, deepening of voice, elevation of mood, and growth of body hair. Hamilton's work also provided an early indication of the potential side-effects of testosterone, or testosterone derivatives; the patient was recorded to have developed acne on his back and chest and experienced hot flushes. Testosterone derivatives are still used to treat this disorder today, although the doses used and the drugs themselves have undergone significant development and modification.

Following the work of Hamilton, a series of reports documented the use of testosterone in the treatment of male involutional melancholia (Barahal, 1938; Danzinger and Blank, 1942; Goldman and Markham, 1942; Davidoff and Goodstone, 1942); this syndrome is believed to be caused by the decrease in testosterone level brought about by the aging process. The research had varying levels of success, but primarily served as a precursor for later research into the application of testosterone-derived treatments in the field of mental health.

In the late 1930s and early 1940s, research was also conducted into the use of testosterone derivatives in the treatment of cardiovascular disorders (Taylor, 1991). Medical and scientific knowledge of today suggests that there is an association between the use and misuse of testosterone and its derivatives and cardiovascular disorders such as myocardial infarction, hypertension and cardiomyopathy (Greenberg *et al.*, 1974; Pearson *et al.*, 1986; Ferenchick, 1990; Ferenchick *et al.*, 1991; Rockhold, 1993; Melchert and Welder, 1995). The use of testosterone as an anti-oestrogen treatment for female breast tumours led to a secondary and more controversial use for testosterone. It has been reported that, during this period, testosterone was administered to homosexual men in the belief that homosexuality was caused by abnormally high levels of female hormones in men (Lenehan *et al.*, 1996).

2.4 The use of testosterone and anabolic steroids for ergogenic purposes

Perhaps the first suggestion that testosterone might be useful in aiding sporting performance came from the work of Oskar Zoth and Fritz Pregl in 1886. As an alternative to testicular transplantation, Zoth and Pregl undertook a study using testicular extracts. These two Austrian scientists aimed to determine whether the aqueous extracts could improve muscle strength and, thus, improve athletic performance. They injected themselves with a liquid extract from bull's testicles and then measured the strength of their middle fingers throughout a series of exercises. Their paper, published in 1896, concluded that the extract had improved the strength and condition of their muscles. Moreover, they went on to suggest that further research be carried out within the athletic community for practical assessment of their initial results. The writer Paul de Kruif reported on the developments in the synthesis and therapeutic applications of testosterone. During the 1940s he commented on the potential of these substances to improve the athletic performance of baseball teams. However, these reports were essentially indications of the potential performance-enhancing abilities of testosterone and its derivatives. The first accurate and controlled studies into this aspect of sports doping were produced in the 1950s.

The American scientist Dr John Ziegler produced some of the most influential work into the effects of AS upon sporting performance. Indeed, Ziegler was responsible for the original synthesis of AS (Taylor, 1991; Goldman and Klatz, 1992; Yesalis *et al.*, 1993a; Hoberman and Yesalis, 1995). In 1956 Ziegler attended the World Games, and at this competition he learnt of the Russian athletes' use of hormonal treatments for perform-ance enhancement. On his return Ziegler reported his findings and, funded by the pharmaceutical company Ciba, went on to synthesize the first AS. He named this compound Dianabol.

Since the development of Dianabol an enormous range of AS has become available. Pharmaceutical companies have continued to research methods to dissociate the 'desirable' anabolic effects from the androgenic effects, but as yet they have had very limited success. Some of the AS available have lower androgenic components than others, but androgenic effects have not been entirely eliminated from any product (Haupt and Rovere, 1984).

The period of the 1960s and 1970s saw an increase in the number of people using AS, and also an increase in the range of AS commercially available (Taylor, 1991). However, the medical and sporting institutions were still viewing these substances with suspicion. In both America and Britain, research as to whether AS did improve athletic performance was conflicting (Johnson and O'Shea, 1968; Freed *et al.*, 1975; Hervey *et al.*, 1976; Ryan, 1978). In 1975, the British Association of Sport and Medicine (BASM) announced that AS were not capable of producing an improvement in performance. The policy of the American College of Sports Medicine (ACSM) was published in their 1977 annual report; this report stated that there was no conclusive scientific evidence to suggest that AS improve athletic performance.

In fact, it was only in the 1980s that it became accepted that, under specified circumstances, AS are capable of producing an improvement in sporting performance. The specific circumstances were that:

the athlete must have been undergoing an intensive weightlifting programme before starting the course of AS;
the athlete must continue this intensive training programme throughout the course of AS;
the athlete must consume a high protein diet.

It also recommended that changes in the strength of the athlete must be measured by the single repetition-maximal weight technique for the exercises in which the athlete trains (Haupt and Rovere, 1984).

After it had become widely accepted that AS could enhance sporting performance, the medical and sporting institutions were forced to change their public policies. The sporting institutions continued to maintain an anti-doping stance. They now had to find some way of deterring athletes from using drugs that were scientifically proven to enhance performance. To compound matters, there was already a significant lack of credibility between the sports medicine and the athletic communities due in no small part to the previous denial of the sport medical community as to the performance-enhancing properties of AS (Haupt and Rovere, 1984). Any research documenting the adverse effects of these drugs was likely to be viewed sceptically by athletes.

2.5 *The use of anabolic steroids in sports*

The use of AS as performance-enhancing drugs among sportsmen spread throughout the world within two decades. Body-builders on the West Coast of America experimented with steroid preparations throughout the late 1940s and early 1950s (Goldman and Klatz, 1992; Yesalis *et al.*, 1993b). Understandably, as stories of their success spread, competitors in other strength-intensive sports began using the drugs to enhance their perform-ance on the track and field. Over the past 40 years, the use of AS has taken place in an increasing number of sports, including football, swimming, cycling, wrestling and many more (Wallechinsky, 1996). Steroid use is even well documented among athletes in college and high school (Buckley *et al.*, 1988; Johnson *et al.*, 1989; Schroff, 1992).

Anabolic steroid users from different sports use different doses of AS. Doses used by endurance athletes tend to be at or below physiologic replace-ment levels, whereas athletes in sports where 'bulk' is desirable, e.g. weight-lifting, use doses far in excess of physiologic levels (Yen and Jaffe, 1978; Francis, 1990; Yesalis, 1993). The close community of many elite-level teams may have influenced the various doses used by different athletes; a swimmer would obviously be less likely to desire the same 'bulkiness' as a weightlifter, or wrestler. It is possible that as AS use spread into the different types of sports, so did advice from more experienced users. Anabolic steroids may be used by athletes to improve their performance in the pre-competition period. The difference between AS as doping agents and other drugs, such as amphetamines or cocaine, is that AS may be used during training sessions to produce improvements, but their use can be ceased before the competition and therefore the chance of detection in drugs tests may be reduced. Anabolic steroids are usually used in cycles. An 'on-cycle' is the number of weeks for which the AS are used; an on-cycle is generally followed by a period of abstinence from AS, or an 'off-cycle'. The length of time for which the individual uses AS tends to be variable, with an average on-cycle lasting from between 8 to 12 weeks and an off-cycle of similar duration (Yesalis, 1993). However, there are reports that some AS users administer AS on a continual basis (Duchaine, 1989; Lenehan *et al.*, 1996). Most of the other doping methods are based entirely on the principle of improving performance on a more short-term basis by drug use immediately before a competiton or event (Goldman and Klatz, 1992).

Tests for AS were developed by Donike in the 1960s; the early tests used a gas chromatography method to detect the presence of AS, and AS metabolites, in urine (Donike and Stratmann, 1974). Athletes that test positive for any substance may face severe penalties and as the tests have progressively become more sophisticated and sensitive, many involved in elite sport have attempted to apply a variety of methods to avoid detection (Voy, 1991; Goldman and Klatz, 1992). The concomitant use of other drugs, such as masking agents, to avoid detection in drugs tests, e.g. Probnecid, or drugs to ameliorate adverse effects of AS has become part of the AS-using culture (Lenehan *et al.*, 1996).

2.6 *The non-competitive use of anabolic steroids*

The use of AS has spread from the circles of elite athletes to include a range of users from diverse backgrounds and occupations (Lenehan *et al.*, 1996), with an increasing number of young people using AS for cosmetic purposes (Melia, 1994). The media trend of male attractiveness, based upon muscularity, may have been related to this extension of prevalence. The promotion of a muscular physique in the popular culture is also stated as a possible cause for the increase in use of AS among adolescents (Komoroski and Rickert, 1992; Faigenbaum *et al.*, 1998).

Numerous studies have reported that very high doses of AS are used by individuals not involved in elite spot (Strauss *et al.*, 1985; Tricker *et al.*, 1989, Williamson and Young, 1992; Korkia *et al.*, 1996, Lenehan *et al.*, 1996). It is also apparent that most of these individuals are using AS without any medical supervision, thus presenting an increased risk to their health (Lenehan *et al.*, 1996). Women and adolescent AS users may be especially at risk of suffering from the adverse effects of AS use when these drugs are taken at high doses (Strauss, 1984).

Lenehan *et al.* (1996) outline three categories of AS users:

1 Professional and serious amateur athletes – the main aim of this group in taking AS is to improve sporting performance.
2 Occupational users – these users take AS with the aim of improving their ability to do their jobs. Individuals that may be represented in this group include manual labourers, or those involved in the entertainment industry.

3 Recreational users (and weight trainers training for cosmetic purposes) – this group uses AS to maintain body weight/physical appearance or to increase libido.

Lenehan noted that the first group of professional and serious amateur athletes is the smallest group of users, although within this community the percentage of users might be higher than in the general population.

A larger number of studies regarding adolescent AS use have been conducted in the USA than in Britain, although there are reasons to believe that the trend for adolescent AS use has already crossed the Atlantic. There are many concerns with regard to adolescent AS use. First, the side-effects that may be experienced by the adolescent AS user are potentially serious. For example, it has been suggested that the use of AS before full height has been attained can result in stunted growth. Several studies suggest that adolescent AS users may be at risk of other problems such as an elevated risk of injury and changes in spermatogenesis (Rosenfeld *et al.*, 1982; Blether *et al.*, 1984; Strauss, 1987; Buckley *et al.*, 1988; Wilson *et al.*, 1988).

Research conducted by the Canadian Centre for Drug Free Sport (Melia, 1994) showed that a higher proportion of the under-18-years age group used AS to improve their appearance rather than to improve their sporting performance. Komoroski and Rickert (1992) studied body image and attitudes to AS use among 1492 adolescents in Arkansas. Their work revealed significant differences between AS users and non-users in risk-taking behaviours, and they showed that AS use was strongly motivated by social influences and knowledge of other AS users.

It is reported that in the 1960s Dianabol was administered to each player in an American high-school football team throughout the season. Anabolic steroids are stated to have been prescribed to these individuals by a medical doctor who was in collaboration with a pharmaceutical company (Gilbert, 1969; Yesalis, 1993). Further reports of doping in adolescents are also stated to have occurred; a study carried out in 1965 documented that tenth- to eleventh-grade football players were administered with three different brands of AS (Gilbert, 1969; Yesalis *et al.*, 1993b). The use of AS by adolescents in the USA may be a result of the intense pressure for high-school and collegiate sports scholarships; parents have been reported to supply their children with AS to improve their child's sporting performance (Kendrick, 1999).

Adolescent AS has a number of implications for society. Many studies have documented the link between AS use and risk-taking behaviour (Komoroski and Rickert, 1992), and other links have been established with use of other illicit substances (Buckley *et al.*, 1988; Johnson, 1990; Schroff, 1992). Work by Yesalis *et al.* (1993b) has shown that 80% of the 12- to 17-years age group involved in their study stated that within the past year they had acted aggressively against people or committed a crime against property.

2.7 *Prevalence studies*

2.7.1 POTENTIAL SOURCES OF ERROR AND MISREPRESENTATION

Most prevalence studies do not present an overall view of the numbers of individuals using AS. A number of difficulties are involved in determining the number of AS users in the population. Many of the past studies have focused on small groups of users from targeted gyms or groups. Studies involving gym users only give an indication of the number of AS users involved in those particular activities, such studies are not representative of a potentially wider population of AS users that do not attend gyms or attend gyms of the type not included in the specific study.

Another source of error in prevalence studies is related to the individuals involved and their honesty in reporting either their own or others' use of steroids. It is well established that in certain situations respondents are likely to either under- or over-report the relevant information. The degree of accuracy of these studies is determined by the honesty of the respondents. Yesalis *et al.* (1993b) estimated that AS users are more likely to under-report the prevalence of AS use and those that do not use AS are more likely to over-report the use of these substances. From these assumptions it is probable that the actual prevalence of AS use lies between the lower limits of the over-reported figures and the upper limits of the statistics most likely to be under-reported. Reasons for these discrepancies in accuracy are numerous, with suggestions that under-reporting may stem from anxiety about drug use being discovered or the unwillingness of the athletic community to discuss doping methods (Dubin, 1990).

It is clear that AS are used by a diverse range of individuals for many different purposes. The use of these substances has expanded into a wider arena where individuals may now be using these drugs for reasons other than enhancement of sporting performance (Lenehan *et al.*, 1996).

2.7.2 PREVALENCE OF AS USE AMONG ADOLESCENTS AND YOUNG PEOPLE

In recent years there has been concern about the number of adolescents and young people starting to use AS. Some of the most in-depth research into the prevalence of AS use within this age group has been conducted in the USA and Canada. However, recent studies in the north-west of England have highlighted the existence of an adolescent AS-using community in Britain. A study involving schoolchildren from the Sefton area of Merseyside (Metropolitan Borough of Sefton, 1998) showed that AS were offered to boys more frequently than any substance other than cannabis and amphetamines.

In this study AS had been offered to 6.4% of the boys and 1.3% of the girls. The percentages of year 10 boys and girls who admitted using AS were 2.4% and 0.2%, respectively.

A study by Lenehan *et al.* (1996) examined the use of AS in gyms across the north-west of England. A total of 24 (N = 386) individuals under the age of 20 years were reported to use AS. Their study also showed that 30% of the total sample first used AS while still teenagers. The youngest age of first use in this study was 15 years. The 1998–1999 First Annual Report and National Plan (The UK Anti-Drugs Co-ordinator, 1998–1999) stated concern that the age of first use of all types of drugs may be getting younger.

The Canadian Centre for Drug Free Sport performed research to establish the prevalence of AS use among Canadian adolescents (Melia *et al.*, 1996). This study involved 16,119 school-aged Canadians from five regions of Canada: 2.8% of the respondents were reported to have used AS in the year before the survey, and 29.4% of these individuals had administered the AS by injection. A number of these individuals reported they had shared needles during their AS use. These figures were extrapolated to provide an estimation that over 83,000 school-aged Canadians had used AS in the 12 months prior to the study.

In the USA, Buckley *et al.* (1988) performed an influential study into the estimated prevalence of AS use among male high-school seniors. This study also showed that certain users start to use AS while under the age of 16 years; over two-thirds of the user group came into this category. The overall results of the study showed that 6.6% of the twelfth-grade males involved had used, or were currently using, AS. A more recent study of adolescent AS use in the USA has shown that adolescent girls are increasing in numbers faster than any other group of users (Yesalis *et al.*, 1997).

Komoroski and Rickert (1992) studied body image and attitudes to AS use among 1492 adolescents in Arkansas. Their work revealed significant differences between AS users and non-users in risk-taking behaviours, and they also showed that AS use was strongly motivated by social influences and knowledge of other AS users. Numerous other studies have been conducted into the prevalence of AS use among adolescents in the USA (Johnson *et al.*, 1989; Elliot and Goldberg, 1996; Kersey, 1996; DuRant *et al.*, 1997; Nutter, 1997; Faigenbaum *et al.*, 1998). Generally these studies show that the prevalence rate for AS use is higher among the male than the female adolescent population (Bahrke *et al.*, 1998).

Studies have shown that use of AS by adolescents is occurring on a global scale. Handelsman and Gupta (1997) studied the AS use of high-school students from a random sample of 203 high schools in New South Wales and Victoria, Australia. A total of 13,555 students, 51.3% of whom were male and with an overall median age of 13.8 years, completed self-report questionnaires. The results indicated that 3.2% of the males and 1.2% of the females had used AS. Factors that were shown to be associated with the use of AS included truancy (for seven or more days over the fortnight prior to questionnaire completion), Aboriginality, speaking only a non-English language at home, having a high student income, and being born overseas.

A study by Lambert *et al.* (1998) revealed similar prevalence rates in their study of 16–18-year-old schoolchildren from two regions of South Africa. Again, the use of AS was more common among males than females. This study additionally investigated the levels of general knowledge, and knowledge about AS, and showed that knowledge levels for both factors were low among AS users. They also discovered that male AS users who were participating in sports experienced a greater pressure to conform than non-AS-using sports participants. This is especially interesting when considering the peer pressure prevalent among adolescents, and the findings from previous research (Salva and Bacon, 1991; Faigenbaum *et al.*, 1998) that adolescent AS use is associated with having friends that use AS.

One of the most disturbing aspects of adolescent use of AS is that previous studies have indicated that young AS users seldom obtain information about AS from reliable medical services (Komoroski and Rickert, 1992; Tanner *et al.*, 1995; Lambert *et al.*, 1998). This may be indicative of a lack of appropriate advice services or a lack of awareness among adolescents about the possible sources of reliable drug information. As mentioned previously, AS use has been frequently associated with use of AS among the individual's group of friends; it may be that adolescent users feel more comfortable with discussing drug issues with their peer group and feel that other sources of advice are inaccessible.

A study in Sweden found that among 15- to 16-year-olds, use was as high as 10%, with 50% of this number injecting AS (Nilsson, 1995). A study of doping among high-school students ($N = 2742$) from the Uppsala region of Sweden showed that 2.7% of the male students and 0.4% of the female students had used performance-enhancing drugs at some stage in their life.

Other factors that have been associated with use of AS among adolescents include participation in strength-related sports and use of other illicit drugs (Bahrke *et al.*, 1998). It is becoming more apparent that young teenagers are attracted to using AS, not to improve athletic performance or strength but just to improve their looks and physique. The increasing macho cult and subtle effects of advertising tempt teenagers to acquire physical attributes normally associated with a more mature figure. The North American experience appears to be slightly different in that there is a greater pressure for adolescents to use AS for a competitive edge, as that society places more of an emphasis on success in sports (Melia, 1994). A study of the perceptions of doping in elite and recreational sport in Switzerland showed that 13 out of 14 parents would not hold back their children from sports, even though they considered doping to be a serious threat to the health and ethics of those involved in sport (Nocelli *et al.*, 1998).

There are other studies regarding adolescent AS use in Sweden (Kindlundh *et al.*, 1998), France (Laure, 1998), England (Lenehan *et al.*, 1996; Metropolitan Borough of Sefton, 1998) and Canada (Melia *et al.*, 1996). It seems that although these countries are diverse, adolescents may experience a common pressure to 'improve' their bodies for reasons such as enhancement of sporting performance or cosmetic factors. Contemporary youth culture is full of images that, it can be argued, exert pressure on adolescents to strive for a body that will give them a more positive image of themselves. Magazines read by young people contain images of male icons. Magazines for both male and female adolescents portray images of semi-naked males with well-developed physiques. Music videos also contain this type of imagery, thus reinforcing the message to young males about the type of body image that they should be striving for as it would be admired by both their peer group and also the young women they hope to impress. Anabolic steroids might be seen as a quick and effective way of escaping the limitations of an adolescent body and progressing to adulthood (Korkia and Stimson, 1993).

2.7.3 PREVALENCE OF AS USE AMONG ADULT FEMALES

Research suggests that a smaller number of adult females use AS than males (Korkia and Stimson, 1993; Lenehan *et al.*, 1996). As yet there are no studies that provide reasons for this difference, and studies regarding the prevalence of AS use among females are scarce. It may be that societal issues such as perceptions of the 'ideal' female body image are related to the lower frequency in the population of female AS users. Other factors that may be related to the lower use of AS may include the reluctance of females to be seen as using methods of doping, particularly those methods, such as use of AS, that are associated with potentially masculinizing side-effects.

Since AS were first synthesized, the roles of women have undergone a series of changes. The 1960s saw a new attitude towards many 'old' values. It is speculated that the first females to use AS for enhancement of sporting performance were elite-level athletes from the Eastern Bloc countries (Yesalis *et al.*, 1993b). Positive tests for AS have been reported for a number of females in sporting competitions (Jennings, 1996; Wallechinsky, 1996). However, studies into use of AS by women are infrequent. The number of women that want to be involved in research might be small as a result of reluctance of women to admit to drug use (Strauss *et al.*, 1985; Korkia *et al.*, 1996), and it might be that this is related to issues of child care and the traditional feminine image (Duda, 1986b).

Conventional and media representations of the 'ideal' female body tend not to be well muscled (Lenskyj, 1986; Cashmore, 1990). Muscles are generally equated with masculinity (Rosenkrantz *et al.*, 1968) and females involved in stereotypically masculine sports are not viewed positively (Kane and Snyder, 1989). However, since the 1960s women's roles have become more varied and the women's movement has been influential in the struggle against the stereotyping of females. Women are now able to compete in a wide variety of sports and to pursue careers that were previously restricted to males.

A range of occupations in which strength and muscularity are desirable have now become viable career options for women. These women are now under the same pressure as men not to be tempted into using AS to improve their ability to perform in their job. Occupations such as the armed forces, in which females may now be in active combat, and the security business, where females may be employed as door staff and security guards, are pertinent examples.

The medical uses of AS in the treatment of women are diverse. These drugs have been used to treat female to male transsexuals (Westaby *et al.*, 1977), and for the treatment of a variety of disorders. Anabolic steroids and other testosterone-derived treatments carry the risk to females of permanent side-effects such as deepening of the voice, clitoral enlargement, increased growth of facial and body hair and reduction in breast size (Strauss *et al.*, 1985; Korkia *et al.*, 1996), and this has led to their limited use in the treatment of women. The principle behind the use of testosterone and testosterone-derived drugs is that these substances may neutralize the effects of oestrogen. Hoberman and Yesalis (1995) report that advertisements for male hormone treatment have been included in medical journals since the early 1920s, when these treatments were used in attempts to alleviate female conditions such as menstrual problems and breast conditions, including tumours.

Testosterone therapy was used to treat women in the 1940s with breast cancer. These treatments are still used today for women suffering from post-menopausal androgen-dependent breast cancer (Hoberman and Yesalis, 1995). A consequence of the research in the 1940s was that it was observed that the testosterone treatment served to increase the women's sex drive, appetite and general feelings of well-being. Testosterone therapies were also used to increase the libido in women, but this type of treatment is not current standard medical practice.

As mentioned previously, the number of adolescent females using AS appears to be increasing at a faster rate than any other group of AS users (Yesalis *et al.*, 1997). Other studies of the prevalence of AS use among adolescents have also documented the use of AS by female adolescents (Handelsman and Gupta, 1997; Faigenbaum *et al.*, 1998; Lambert *et al.*, 1998). This is particularly worrying because this group of users may be at a high risk of developing adverse symptoms as a consequence of their AS use, some of which may be irreversible, such as deepening of the voice and clitoral enlargement (Strauss *et al.*, 1985). It has been claimed that females are more sensitive to AS than males (Buckley *et al.*, 1988); the basis of this claim stems from the fact that AS are derivatives of the male hormone testosterone, and this hormone is responsible for the development and main-tenance of male secondary sexual characteristics and is found only in very small amounts in women.

Korkia and Stimson (1997) conducted a prevalence study involving 21 gyms in England, Scotland and Wales. They found that 2.3% of the women ($N = 1667$) had used AS in the past and 1.4% were currently using AS. A study of AS use in the north-west of England (Lenehan *et al.*, 1996) showed that of the 386 respondents interviewed, all of whom were attending gyms in the area studied, seven were women. This is a small percentage of the total number of AS users, although it is representative only of those women that admitted to using AS. All of these women were involved in competitive body-building.

Body-building is frequently perceived to be a sport closely related to the use of AS (Ryan, 1981; Duda, 1986b; Tricker *et al.*, 1989), and public perceptions of body-builders tend to be varied (Klein, 1984; Kane, 1988). The first female body-building competition was held in 1977 in Ohio, USA (Duff and Hong, 1984), and female body-building competitions are now held in many countries around the world. There are a limited number of studies about female body-builders but 'underground' steroid handbooks, generally written by and for those involved in the AS-using culture, seem to suggest that AS use is not restricted to male body-builders (Duchaine, 1989; Hart, 1993). Often these texts suggest that women use lower doses of AS than men.

A study of needle exchanges in the Merseyside and Cheshire regions of England showed that the number of female AS users attending needle-exchange schemes had decreased between 1992 and 1996 (Birtles, 1998). This reduction in attendance presents a cause for concern as it may be representative of women feeling excluded from drug agencies. However, it may also reflect a reduction in the number of females using AS. Awiah *et al.* (1990) have also reported that many women drug users are reluctant to attend drug agencies. Studies have shown that certain females do inject AS (Strauss *et al.*, 1985; Korkia *et al.*, 1996), and thus the needle-exchange figures may be a misrepresentation of the actual numbers of females injecting AS.

2.7.4 PREVALENCE OF AS USE AMONG ADULT MALES

Use of AS by males seems to be more prevalent globally than among females. Many of the studies into the effects of AS have focused almost entirely upon male subjects (Buckley *et al.*, 1988; Su *et al.*, 1993; Cooper *et al.*, 1996). Statistics for the prevalence of AS use among males in the UK suggest that an estimated 9% of males attending gyms have used AS (Korkia and Stimson, 1993). In the USA, Yesalis *et al.* (1993b) used data from the 1991 National Household survey on Drug Use to perform a national study of prevalence of AS use. From a total of 32,594 respondents 0.9% of the males (compared to 0.1% of females) had used AS at some stage of their lives. Also in the USA, a study involving over 1600 college athletes was conducted to estimate the level of their competitors' AS use (Yesalis *et al.*, 1993b). The mean overall projected rate of any prior use of AS across all sports surveyed was 14.7% for male athletes and 5.9% for female athletes.

A study of the prevalence of drug use among Finnish male prisoners was conducted by Korte *et al.* in 1995. This study was undertaken at four prisons, where 354 prisoners responded to the survey; 3.7% of the respond-ents stated they had taken AS while in their current prison. Prisoners aged 25 years and younger were found to have a significantly higher rate of drug use. As yet, similar studies of prison populations in the UK have not been carried out. However, the Finnish study suggests that AS use may be pre-valent even in the controlled environment of prisons.

Male body-builders have been frequently associated with AS use (O'Connor, 1995). Various studies have shown that use of AS occurs at the competitive, amateur and recreational levels (Tricker *et al.*, 1989; Delbeke *et al.*, 1995; Lenehan *et al.*, 1996). It is perhaps important to mention that the discovery of AS use by a recreational or amateur body-builder may be less damaging, in terms of the implications on the career and financial situation of the individual involved, than it would be to a professional/elite-level athlete. In a study of AS use in the north-west of England it was found that the greatest proportion of the sample ($N = 386$) was involved in competitive or recreational body-building (94.5% in total), whereas the number of AS users involved in competitive sport was considerably lower (1.8%) (Lenehan *et al.*, 1996). Although this does not provide conclusive evidence that AS use is more preval-ent in body-building than in competitive sport, it does suggest that converse to public perception (Nocelli *et al.*, 1998), doping methods are apparent in amateur and recreational sports, and not restricted to elite-level sport.

2.7.5 PREVALENCE OF AS USE AMONG ELITE ATHLETES

The small size of this community and its regular participation in drugs tests would lead many to believe that it should be easier to obtain relatively accurate prevalence data. However, despite these preconceptions it may in fact be more difficult to assess the prevalence of AS use in this community than in other populations. Severe penalties are imposed by the International Olympic Committee (IOC) and many other sporting bodies if the use of AS is detected. The penalties of a positive drugs test may also have serious repercussions for the public image and financial situation of the athletes and their sport. For these reasons it may be difficult to get AS-using athletes to admit to their drug use, and to give honest responses to questions about the drug use within their area of sport. It is also difficult to rely on the number of positive drugs tests to determine prevalence of AS use. A variety of methods have been used by athletes to avoid detection in drugs tests. The use of masking agents, catheterization of urine, sample substitution and sample manipulation are just a few of the methods previously used (Voy, 1991; Mottram, 1996).

An additional difficulty encountered when relying upon positive drug test results to indicate prevalence rates for AS use is related to the way in which these substances are used. Anabolic steroids may be used during pre-competition training periods, and if the athlete ceases to use these substances in enough time before a competition drug test detection they may avoid the detection of illicit substances (Goldman and Klatz, 1992). Thus, the positive drug test data do not provide an overall view of the use of AS among the athletic community (Dubin, 1990). It has been suggested that out-of-competition drug testing may combat this type of behaviour. However, the success of out-of-competition testing in reducing the international spread of AS use in sport depends upon international co-operation. If certain countries are proceeding with out-of-competition testing when others are not, there could be difficulties in maintaining fair competition at international sporting events. Other difficulties in the implementation of such a strategy are related to the diligence with which each country implements this type of testing regime. The financial burdens that may be created by such a scheme could present difficulties for Third-World or developing countries. This problem was highlighted as early as 1990 when the Dubin Report (1990) suggested that perhaps Canada should not compete against countries where out-of-competition testing did not occur. It also suggested that the International Amateur Athletic Federation (IAAF) should provide financial support to countries in which out-of-competition testing may be difficult to conduct because of technical difficulties and financial costs.

A study of the prevalence of doping in sports in Norway from 1977 to 1995 (Bahr and Tjornhom, 1998) showed that an increase in the frequency of doping tests was associated with a decrease in the percentage of positive samples in targeted sports. This study involved a total of 15,208 athletes, most of whom belonged to national federations under the jurisdiction of the Norwegian Confederation of Sport (NCS), and it is interesting to note that 90% of the tests performed were unannounced.

In the past, AS have been frequently associated with strength-dependent sports such as weightlifting and wrestling. It has been suggested that certain athletes may use AS in the belief that this is the only way in which they can compete with drug-using competitors (Heikkala, 1993; Black and Pape, 1997). It would be logical to assume that this type of drug use may be self-perpetuating in that participants in sports previously associated with a high prevalence of AS use are more likely to use AS for this reason. However, the use of AS is not exclusive to these types of sports, and reports of AS use by swimmers, cyclists and sprinters have been frequent (George, 1996a; Verroken, 1996). Some of the potential effects of AS use are clearly more beneficial to certain sports than others. Thus it would be expected that the prevalence rates for AS use in sports such as figure skating, where high muscle mass, or 'bulk', is not a crucial factor for success, might be less than in the more conventional strength sports such as weightlifting (Yen and Jaffe, 1978; Francis, 1990).

The actual prevalence rates of AS use among elite athletes are believed to be high (Dubin, 1990). In a testimony about the use of AS by US athletes between the 1984 and 1988 Olympics, Pat Connolly declared that at least 40% of the women's team in Seoul had probably used steroids at some time in their preparations for the games. This again highlights the issue of out-of-competition use of AS.

A prevalence study of powerlifters in the USA (Curry and Wagman, 1999) reviewed the use of AS among 28 members of teams of US powerlifters. Of the 15 members that returned the postal questionnaires, 10 admitted using AS, and five admitted they had evaded the IOC's doping control procedures while using AS.

Scarpino *et al.* (1990) carried out research about the prevalence of doping among Italian athletes. Their work involved 1015 Italian athletes and 216 coaches, doctors and managers. Results showed that over 10% of the athletes admitted to frequent use of AS at national- and international-level sport. It is interesting that 62% of the athletes that acknowledged doping stated that there was pressure from coaches and managers to use doping methods to improve performance. The research also stated that 70% of the athletes felt that access to illegal substances was easy.

2.7.6 THE INDICATIONS FOR PREVALENCE OF AS USE IN THE UK

At present, accurate statistics for prevalence of AS use in the UK are not available. As mentioned earlier, there are many variables that may render small- or large-scale prevalence studies inaccurate. Previous British studies, such as those by Lenehan *et al.* (1996) of AS use in the north-west of England and the Williamson (1993) study of drug use at a technical college in Stirling, provide only localized information. It is perhaps easier, and possibly more practical, for us to consider the trends and patterns of AS use rather than simply the number involved in this type of behaviour. In this way we may be better equipped to understand and alleviate any of the problems stemming from this type of substance use. The importance of factors such as availability of fake or counterfeit steroids, use of clean injecting equipment and regular medical checks for users should also be considered.

Korkia and Stimson (1993) attempted to explore the extent and uses of AS in the UK from a public health perspective. Twenty-one gymnasia in England, Scotland and Wales were surveyed by questionnaire yielding a response rate of 59% (1667 respondents). They found that 9.1% of men and 2.3% of women had taken AS at some time, and 6% of men and 1.4% of women were current users. Considerable variation was found in the prevalence of use, ranging from no reports (in three gyms) to 46%. Patterns of use and perceived side-effects were investigated with a group of 110 AS users recruited through social networks.

In-depth interviews with the users revealed that 97 men and 13 women had been using AS regularly for 2.05 and 1.9 years, respectively. Seventy-two of those interviewed injected AS. Up to 16 different drugs were taken by interviewees during the present or last cycle. Most (77%) interviewees reported experiencing two or more side-effects. Of the 97 men interviewed, 56% reported testicular atrophy, 52% gynaecomastia, 36% elevated blood pressure, 56% fluid retention, 25% injuries to tendons, 22% nosebleeds and 16% frequent colds. Six men reported problems with kidney function and five with liver function. Of the 13 women interviewed, eight reported menstrual irregularities, eight fluid retention, four clitoral enlargement, three decreased breast size, and two elevated blood pressure. Forty-eight per cent were concerned about the long-term side-effects of AS use, and 44% indicated that they would discontinue taking AS if it were proven that they could cause serious side-effects, such as cancer. Twenty-two per cent indicated that they would not stop using AS and 33% were unsure. Fifteen per cent reported having permanent side-effects. Eighty-seven per cent said that they would continue using AS even if their possession became illegal. Over a third (35%) said that they received regular medical checks for AS use. Although the data from this study do not attempt to estimate the number of AS users in the UK, it does suggest that AS use is relatively common among regular gym attenders in British towns. The results suggest that AS use has diffused in many parts of Britain, with 'pockets' of very high-user groups. The authors state that it is impossible to estimate the prevalence for Britain as there are no reliable data regarding the number of gyms in the UK.

Lenehan *et al.* (1996) used a similar method to Korkia and Stimson, except that they included more types of gymnasia (*n* = 43), and used trusted outreach workers to administer the survey; this might explain the higher level of AS use reported. Of 58% responding, 50% of hardcore (respondents mostly using freestanding weights) users, 31% of mixed (more strength than cardiovascular equipment) users and 13% of fitness (more cardiovascular than strength equipment) users reported that they had taken AS.

Perry *et al.* (1992) conducted a prevalence study of AS use among people using gymnasia on a regular basis (i.e. three or more times a week) in West Glamorgan. The rate of use was 38.8% out of 160 individuals. Over 58% of AS users admitted injecting more than 30 times, and 57% of injectors admitted to injecting in the year prior to interview. Fifty per cent had taken oral AS in the previous year and 56.4% had taken tablets on 30 or more occasions. The potential for HIV transmission via needle sharing was a particular concern in this study. Eight people had been involved in some form of needle-sharing activity.

2.8 Needle and syringe exchange figures for prevalence of AS use

The National Forum for Drug Data (NFDD), a body prepared by the Drug Misuse Database Managers and the Department of Health, undertook a study of the, then, 14 regional databases to discover the level and standard-ization of data collection from syringe exchange schemes (SES) around the country. Eight collected some data from at least some SES in their area but the quality would appear to be variable. Those who did not collect data from SES stated that the main reasons were lack of resources and problems with the data, awaiting a nationally agreed methodology. SES data are not col-lected everywhere and where they are collected there is not a standard dataset (Birtles, 1998). This prevents the assessment of the nationwide picture of SES use and AS presentations in particular. Such a dataset would be able to inform a comprehensive study, which should also include data gathered from gyms and GPs, police and Customs.

Anecdotally, more users are using SES equipment than are seen at SES and are getting it via an advocate, that is one person will go to an SES and acquire injecting equipment for a number of colleagues. Also large numbers of AS users are purchasing injecting equipment from their dealers. Thus, despite the significantly high numbers of AS users presenting to services, this may just be the tip of the iceberg.

The following data come from the Drug Misuse Database for Merseyside (J. McVeigh, personal communication). They show that new AS users now outnumber opiate users. This will obviously have an effect on the service being provided to the core clients of the service, the opiate users. It is also interesting to note the reduction in heroin users attending the service, as this might be related to the increase in the number of AS users. There is no other indication that heroin use is slowing down in this area. Anecdotally, there is a certain animosity between opiate users attending syringe-exchange services and opiate users as AS users do not see themselves as drug users in the conventional sense. They can be disparaging to these users, seeing them-selves as different from the 'smack heads' or 'junkies' that use the same syringe-exchange services. This in itself would seem to suggest that there is a need to provide some level of dedicated services for AS users.

Main drug of use	Number of new clients attending agency-based syringe exchange in Mersey 1998–2001			
	1998	1999	2000	2001
Heroin	549	536	472	498
Methadone	46	26	25	21
Amphetamine	76	59	12	18
Steroids	**398**	**469**	**469**	**558**
Cocaine	27	27	15	12
Other	31	43	40	21

2.9 *Social implications of the psychological effects of AS use*

Anabolic steroids are associated with a range of adverse side-effects. Some of the adverse symptoms linked with AS are classified as psychological, or psychiatric. From the mid-1980s onwards the popular press has been reporting the incidence of rages induced by AS, termed 'roid rages' (Lubell, 1989). There has been a significant level of controversy regarding the influence that AS may have upon the judgement of the individual user. Anabolic steroids have been associated with a number of violent crimes (Lubell, 1989; Lenehan *et al.*, 1996); however, there has been speculation regarding the amount of influence these drugs exerted upon the offender's behaviour. It is interesting to note that although AS are now associated with adverse psychological symptoms, they were used between the 1930s and the mid-1980s, with varying levels of success, in the treatment of psychological disorders, such as depression (Taylor, 1991).

Research into the psychological effects of illicit AS use is difficult because it is more or less impossible to replicate the conditions under which AS are used illicitly. However, Su *et al.* (1993) conducted research into the effects of high doses of AS. They found that men taking a high dose of AS were likely to experience effects that included increased irritability, increased violent tendencies, increased mood swings and an increase in anger. This study was controlled and double blind, the subjects were also screened for previous substance misuse and psychological problems before taking part in the study. Other studies have shown similar relationships between use of AS and changes in mood and behaviour (Pope and Katz, 1988; Kouri *et al.*, 1995; Corrigan, 1996; Lenehan *et al.*, 1996; Borowsky *et al.*, 1997).

It has also been suggested that some users of AS have a predisposition towards personality disorders. Cooper *et al.* (1996) conducted a study that showed that one in three of the AS-using individuals in their research satisfied the diagnostic criteria for at least one of the personality disorders before they started to use AS. These included paranoid, schizotypal, antisocial, borderline, histrionic, narcissistic, and passive–aggressive personality trait disorders. Their results also suggested that significant disturbances in personality profile are associated with, and possibly a direct result of, AS use. A study by Porcerelli and Sandler (1995) outlined a positive relationship between narcissistic personality traits and use of AS. Their study compared two groups made up of weightlifters and body-builders, one group consisting of AS users, the other of non-AS users. The AS-using group had significantly lower levels of empathy but significantly higher levels of narcissism than the non-AS-using group. The only difficulty involved in the interpretation of these results stems from the fact that personality traits prior to onset of AS use were not recorded, therefore it is impossible to conclude whether a predisposition to such traits is related to the initiation of AS use.

It is interesting that in a study of general practitioners from the Liverpool, Birmingham and Berkshire areas of the UK, the largest number of adverse effects observed by the doctors were psychological/psychiatric in nature. This result was common to all three areas surveyed (Lenehan *et al.*, unpublished).

The potential societal implications of these adverse psychological effects have been documented in a number of reports. Murder (Dalby, 1992; Corrigan, 1996), armed robbery (Dalby, 1992), domestic violence (Schulte *et al.*, 1993; Choi and Pope, 1994; Stanley and Ward, 1994) and child abuse (Schulte *et al.*, 1993) are examples of crimes that have been associated with abuse of AS. The effects of AS and testosterone derivatives upon road aggression are also subject to research. Ellingrod *et al.* (1997) conducted a study using the Iowa driving simulator to discover the effects of physiologic and supraphysiologic doses of testosterone cypionate. They used weekly doses of 100 mg, 250 mg and 500 mg, and then tested the driving behaviour of the subjects. The study did not provide conclusive evidence of a relationship between AS and aggressive driving behaviour, but it was suggested that greater doses of testosterone cypionate, i.e. over 500 mg per week, may be responsible for alterations in driving behaviour. Further research is required to determine the prevalence of AS-related incidents of driving aggression.

A report by Lubell (1989) documented two murder cases that were associated with AS use, namely the trials of Horace Williams and Glenn Wollstrum. In both cases the men that committed the murders were stated to have been psychologically normal before they started to use AS. At each of the trials the defendants pleaded not guilty because AS use had caused insanity; however, these pleas were rejected by the respective juries and a guilty verdict was passed on both occasions. Although it has been established that use of AS may render certain individuals more prone to aggressive behaviour (Su *et al.*, 1993), there is no conclusive evidence to support the theory that AS can be the direct cause of violence (Lubell, 1989; Pope and Katz, 1990; Kouri *et al.*, 1995).

Research by Choi and Pope (1994) has suggested there is a link between male aggression towards women and AS use. Their study involved AS-using and non-AS-using athletes. The results showed that, while using AS, the user group reported significantly greater levels of aggression towards their female partners. The levels of aggression of the control group of non-AS-using athletes and the AS-using group during their off-drug cycle were not significantly different.

Other research has been carried out to discover the relationship between AS use and sexual aggression. Yates *et al.* (1999) performed a study of the psychosexual effects of testosterone cycling in men. The doses used in this study were 100 mg, 250 mg and 500 mg of testosterone cypionate administered in weekly intramuscular injections. Their work showed that doses of testosterone up to five times the physiologic replacement dose do not present a significant risk of adverse psychosexual effects in most normal men. The study also revealed that at doses starting from 500 mg of testosterone cypionate per week, a small proportion of men are more likely to experience adverse psychosexual effects. This result is particularly interesting because AS users frequently use doses of AS that are significantly greater than the recommended therapeutic dose (Duchaine, 1989; Hart, 1993; Lenehan *et al.*, 1996). A study of sexual aggression in adolescents (Borowsky *et al.*, 1997) has also shown a relationship between use of AS and sexual aggression.

Another particularly important issue is that there may be other drugs used in conjunction with AS; for example, the use of stimulants such as cocaine or amphetamines has been shown to be highly correlated with self-reported aggressive behaviour (The Brown University Digest of Addiction Theory and Application, 1994; Yesalis *et al.*, 1993a). This pattern of drug use is not an uncommon practice in the AS-using community (DuRant *et al.*, 1993; Lenehan *et al.*, 1996; Lukas, 1996).

2.10 *Current therapeutic applications of anabolic steroids*

The therapeutic use of AS has a number of aspects. They may be used with the main aim of changing the levels of hormones, or for the purposes of increasing protein synthesis (Wright, 1978). Since AS were first synthesized there have been developments in the understanding of these drugs. Research into the side-effects of these drugs has led to re-evaluation of their uses; for example, it is now unheard of to use this range of drugs in the treatment of psychological disorders (Taylor, 1991). It has been suggested that, although AS are associated with certain risks, selected patients may find these risks to be acceptable; examples of possible cases include patients with advanced illness or muscle-wasting disease, or patients who have had no success with other treatments (Dobs, 1999).

The American Medical Association (AMA) claim that AS have limited medical uses in the following areas:

1 as treatment of persistent anaemia where red blood cells are unable to regenerate;
2 for control of metastatic breast cancer;
3 for hereditary angio-oedema;
4 to help to stimulate production of plasmin, which helps to break down the protein fibrin – build-up of which can cause thrombosis. These drugs have also been used in other vascular disorders such as Raynaud's syndrome;
5 to assist protein build-up in those weakened after surgery or through long-term confinement;

6 to treat menopausal symptoms – in small doses and in conjunction with the female hormone oestrogen;

7 to replace testosterone in those men who have had the testes removed following surgery for testicular cancer. The prescribing of oral AS in these circumstances helps to maintain the patient's secondary sexual characteristics;

8 to treat adolescent males with pituitary malfunction when they reach the appropriate age for puberty. Anabolics given for 4 to 6 months in the proper dosing schedule cause the growth spurt and development of secondary sexual characteristics.

The AMA admits to being more uncertain about some of these applications than others (such as adjunct therapy for conditions of protein deficiency), but acknowledges that steroids induce a sense of well-being in patients, stimulate the appetite and may be helpful for terminal patients.

The British National Formulary, produced jointly by the British Medical Association and the Royal Pharmaceutical Society, is far more cautious in its view of the medical value of AS. The only positive indication is for aplastic anaemia; the 2001 edition comments: 'Their [AS] protein-building property led to the hope that they might be widely useful in medicine, but this hope has not been realised'. This means that prescribing levels for the drug are low in the UK.

Anabolic steroids have been used to treat individuals with subnormal levels of hormones (Wright, 1978; Taylor, 1991). This application of testosterone therapy has been used in the treatment of impotent males and to initiate the onset of puberty in developmentally delayed boys (Hoberman and Yesalis, 1995). Testosterone derivatives and AS have also been used for their androgenic effects in the treatment of female to male transsexuals (Korkia *et al.*, 1996; Westaby *et al.*, 1977).

Current research is taking place regarding the use of androgen therapy for the treatment of aging in males (Hoberman and Yesalis, 1995). The testosterone-derived treatments are already being used in a London clinic to treat males going through a 'mid-life crisis'. There is speculation that, just as the female menopause has been recognized as a treatable medical complaint, it may be possible to restore the vigour of middle-aged men going through the andropause.

There are a diverse range of medical complaints in which it may be necessary, or desirable, to induce an increase in lean body mass; examples may include people suffering from wasting disease, malnutrition, or other advanced serious illness (Wright, 1978). Anabolic steroids and testosterone derivatives have proved to be effective in the treatment of a number of these types of conditions (Dobs, 1999). Anabolic steroids have been used in cases of malnutrition, including in patients with general non-specific malnutrition. Elderly patients suffering from insufficient dietary protein intake may be prescribed AS to restore their nitrogen balance, increase appetite and muscle mass, and so produce a weight gain (Wright, 1978). Conditions such as cirrhosis, anaemia and pulmonary disease may also benefit from treatment with AS (Mendenhall *et al.*, 1995; Schols *et al.*, 1995; Ferreira *et al.*, 1998). The anabolic effects of AS have also proved to be effective in patients with severe burns (Demling, 1999; Dobs, 1999), and in surgical situations to improve the patients' pre- and postoperative condition (Wright, 1978).

Some of the most recent research into the therapeutic applications of testosterone derivatives and AS has been related to their use in the treatment of patients with HIV. Anabolic steroids have been shown to increase the lean mass and appetite of patients suffering from the muscle-wasting effects of the progression of HIV infection and AIDS (Dobs, 1999; Strawford *et al.*, 1999).

2.11 *Legal status of anabolic steroids*

Anabolic steroids have different legal statuses in different parts of the world. In Britain, AS became subject to the control of The Misuse of Drugs Act on 1 November 1996. They are now categorized as class C drugs and possible penalties for offences are 5 years imprisonment, or an unlimited fine, or both. These restrictions mean that although it is legal to possess AS in quantities for personal use, it is illegal to produce, to supply, or to possess, import or export with intent to supply these substances, without the authority to do so. However, the legislation is vague with regard to the quantities of AS that are deemed as dealer amounts.

In other countries across the world it is still possible to purchase AS legally 'over the counter'. As yet there is limited research comparing the prevalence of AS use between countries where AS are available over the counter and countries where the drugs have to be obtained illicitly and it is unknown whether there are any significant differences between the patterns of AS use.

The USA has an entirely different system of legislation regarding AS. In the USA, AS are classified as schedule III controlled substances under federal law (Taylor, 1991). This legislation was introduced in 1990 as a result of concerns about the health implications of AS use. This legislation means that it is illegal to distribute AS or to possess with intent to distribute AS without a valid prescription. In the USA, the manufacture, distribution, importation, exportation and dispensing of AS is controlled by the Drug Enforcement Administration.

2.12 *Anabolic steroids: a social problem?*

The popular image of the use of doping substances remains focused on sports people and on use in gyms. Increasingly, concern is being expressed that the use of doping substances may be gaining popularity in other settings. Some studies have suggested that homosexual men and young fashion-conscious individuals may be encouraged to use these substances for cosmetic purposes (Korkia and Stimson, 1993).

Commenting on the health risks associated with doping substances is problematic, although I will attempt this in the next chapter. Very few good epidemiological data exist. The range of health effects associated with AS use range from cosmetic changes to more serious and potentially life-threatening conditions. There is therefore an urgent need to identify what is known about the risk of health consequences resulting from the use of doping substances. Such information is of paramount importance in the design of educational material and for ensuring that interventions effectively target high-risk behaviours.

Considerable concern exists about the risks associated with the injection of AS and associated drugs. The context in which injections occur is likely to influence both the risks associated with the behaviour and the public health interventions that are likely to be appropriate (Best and Midgely, 1999).

One of the main observations that can be made from a review of the literature (Haupt and Rovere, 1984; Brower *et al.*, 1994; Yesalis and Cowart, 1998) on the use of AS is how poorly understood are both the social implications and the epidemiology in comparison with other forms of drug consumption (Shapiro, 1992).

This is a concern because the prevalence of use of doping substances and involvement in illicit drug supply is found among certain groups such as night-club security staff and this may represent an opportunity for crossover between the growing illicit drugs market and the market for AS (Maycock, 1999). The patterns of use are often complex, involving multiple substances taken in sophisticated regimes. It is also important to realise that the use of these drugs does not necessarily carry with it the same negative connotations and social stereotypes as the use of other illicit substances. It also remains unclear what will be the most effective strategies for reducing the use of these drugs or reducing the associated harms.

Anabolic steroid use can be viewed as a public policy issue. Public policy making is commonly depicted in terms of a natural logical sequence. From this perspective information about a troubling social issue is highlighted and then documented. It then becomes the role of public policy makers to assess the problem and its causes and to respond to the problem using policy tools such as initiating or adapting laws to deal with the issue. They would then continue to respond to the issue until it was alleviated. This is called the 'rationality perspective' and is the type of process that the public would expect to be in place to deal with social and health problems such as AS misuse (Rochfort and Cobb, 1994).

However, this somewhat simplistic approach does not appear to be mirrored in reality. Dery (1984) states that problems do not simply exist, they are not 'objective entities in their own right'. Rational decision making rarely exists in reality. However, the model remains important as it allows researchers to identify barriers to rational decision making. It is often factors other than the objective conditions that are responsible for an issue's place in the policy makers' hierarchy. These factors will include the intensity of the issue, advocacy and the relevance of competing issues. How does this apply to the issue of AS use?

Traditionally, the use of performance-enhancing drugs (PEDs) has been seen as an issue affecting sport alone. Its depiction in the media generally revolves around major sporting events such as the Olympic games or occasions when sportspeople have tested positive for a banned substance. These flurries of media coverage rarely address the social impact of AS use or the health risks to the wider population. The issue of PEDs, therefore, remains firmly focused within a sporting context in the public consciousness.

There are many perceptions of any particular problem and its place in the public consciousness (Peters and Marshall, 1993). It is only relatively recently that 'problem definition' has been studied as a means of trying to pull together all of the threads that have an impact on issue identification and policy formulation. Decision makers do not see problems in isolation but in a policy context. This involves a number of policies on related issues. The perceived problems may have generated a continually changing set of policies that have evolved over a period of time. In the case of AS and related substances, it is firmly placed in the context of existing drug policy. Therefore, any investigation into the position of AS in a policy context must also look at how it fits into present-day drug policy.

It is difficult to place AS within the UK's drug policy agenda. This is partly because in the early part of the 1990s drug policy was dominated by reducing or preventing the spread of viral infections, such as HIV, by intravenous drug injectors (Advisory Council on the Misuse of Drugs (ACMD), 1988, 1989, 1993). Anabolic steroids did not feature prominently because little research had been done on the extent of AS use and the fact that AS is not injected intravenously. However, some commentators were able to foresee problems related to the transmission of viral infections connected with AS use (Scott and Scott, 1989; Nemechek, 1991). In the latter part of the 1990s drug policy became driven by crime and criminality (Stimson, 2000). Although there has been an association made between AS use and violence (Choi *et al.*, 1990; Schulte *et al.*, 1993), no research has as yet identified an association with AS use and acquisitive crime. The use of AS has therefore not appeared to rate a high position in the current drug policy agenda.

The only attempt by central government to address the issue of the use of AS and other performance-enhancing drugs was the change in the legal status in 1996. There are concerns that the laws could have pushed AS use further underground. Since the legislation was introduced there does not seem to be a slow down in the number of AS users in the UK; in fact the opposite seems to be true. There have been no attempts by the government to educate users or potential users of AS about the dangers inherent in their use or even to provide health professionals with information or guidance not only about the legislation but also about the health issues and treatment of AS users. If this has been an attempt to legislate the issue away, it has obviously failed.

It may be that in future one of the factors influencing the provision of services will be the sheer number of users and the potential for the spread of infections such as HIV. As has been described previously, the number of AS users attending needle exchanges has grown steadily over the past decade. If this trend continues, and it shows no sign of slowing down, then it may be that it is more cost-effective to provide separate services for AS users than dilute and place a strain on the existing services designed for opiate users.

CHAPTER 3

The medical aspects of AS misuse

Anabolic steroids exert multiple actions affecting both the body's organs and its physiology. The results of AS used in animal studies comprise the basis for most of the conclusions concerning the development of side-effects in humans. Rats subjected to levels of AS equivalent to illicit AS use in humans had a dramatically reduced life expectancy (Bronson and Matherne, 1997). Autopsy revealed hepatocytic carcinomas, peliosis hepatis, mesenchymal kidney tumours, lymphosarcomas, pulmonary adenomas and pronounced left ventricular myocardial hypertrophy associated with stenosis of the left atrio-ventricular valve in rats. However, this form of clinical data does not always have significance when applied to humans, as the occurrence of an illness or disease in one species does not mean this will also occur in another.

The most extensive research in humans of side-effect profiles has been in those treated with AS due to severe medical illnesses. Again, it is difficult to apply these clinical findings with any degree of certainty to 'healthy' individuals who use AS. The medical literature comprises mostly single case reports and does not prove a link between cause and effect and it is possible that the individuals concerned may have developed the illness in the absence of AS.

The incidence of death or life-threatening diseases associated with AS use so far has been relatively low and has largely been linked with long-term and high-dose use. Although it may well be that the occurrence of life-threatening events really are rare, it is also possible that such side-effects do not get reported because AS use is probably not considered by practitioners and patients do not always volunteer this information (Lloyd *et al.*, 1996). Short-term effects of AS, such as the derangement of lipid profile, altered liver function and reproductive problems, are well described in the literature. Most of these are reversible with cessation of use, but little reliable information is available about whether or, perhaps more appropriately, at what rate these will translate into life-threatening conditions with long-term or continual use of high dosages and several types of drugs taken together. It is possible that their effects are only realized later in life.

The research that has been conducted has usually been in groups of AS users who have been using their own regimes of drugs, with subjects using different types of AS and dosages. Therefore, no single AS can be individually analysed and any findings in the research have to be applied to the generic group of drugs termed anabolic steroids. As polydrug use among AS users is common, it can be difficult to prove conclusively a direct cause-and-effect relationship between AS use and the disease process.

3.1 *Myocardial hypertrophy and cardiomyopathy*

Skeletal muscle obviously develops strength and mass after periods of weight training and exercise. The heart can also increase in size as the same exercises will cause the heart to work harder in supplying oxygenated blood to the working muscles. Hypertrophy of skeletal and heart muscle is a result of increased protein synthesis due to this repeated resistance loading, but stimulation is by two different mechanisms. Skeletal muscle mass is increased by creating resistance with overloading (e.g. weight training) and cardiac mass is increased by the additional after-load created by the arterial system blood pressure surges that are produced during such exercises (Freedson *et al.*, 1984).

The exogenous use of AS increases the size of skeletal muscle but it is not proven that AS can produce the same effect on heart muscle (Salke *et al.*, 1985). Most studies using echocardiograms to monitor the size of the heart in AS users have found no differences between AS users and with those who train and do not use steroids (Thompson *et al.*, 1992). There was normal growth of septal and left ventricle heart walls but no changes in ventricular chamber size or disproportionate septal thickness. It is apparent that the increase in heart size with exercise is merely a proportional rise with the gain in skeletal muscle bulk (Longhurst *et al.*, 1980) and the exogenous use of steroids does not potentiate the effect of training on heart size (Zuliani *et al.*, 1988). One study of 14 body-builders found that there was enlargement and thickening of the left ventricle but this was not significantly different from the 14 controls (De Piccoli, 1991).

Although studies reporting the results of echocardiography on patients have found no adverse effects, there have been a number of single case reports of cardiomyopathy in the presence of AS use (Ferenchick *et al.*, 1991). Under laboratory conditions, studies of AS *in vitro* have been shown to injure heart muscle, affecting heart rhythm (Melchert *et al.*, 1992). They also cause damage to the cell organelle, mitochondria and cardiac myofibres (Behrendt and Boffin, 1977).

It is believed that AS impairs left ventricular diastolic filling, which may be an early sign of cardiomyopathy (Pearson *et al.*, 1986), and there have been many case reports of sudden death attributed to this (McKillop *et al.*, 1986; Kennedy and Lawrence, 1993). In true hypertrophic obstructive cardiomyopathy there are small ventricular chambers and a forward motion of the mitral valve during systole with early aortic valve closure. These changes are not found in the echocardiograms of body-builders or athletes with hypertrophy of the left ventricular wall (Menapace *et al.*, 1982).

Cardiomyopathy can lead to sudden unexpected death, which, although rare, did occur in young populations even before the widespread use of AS. Post-mortem examination of 29 non-AS-using athletes found that the most common abnormality was hypertrophic cardiomyopathy (Maron *et al.*, 1980), and in a further study of 22 athletes, right ventricular cardiomyopathy was the most prevalent cause of death (Corrado *et al.*, 1990). Enlarged heart size can, therefore, be caused solely by intensive training schedules, but the problem may be compounded by the administration of exogenous hormones. Thibilin *et al.* (2000) describes the results of autopsies on 34 male AS users that were conducted for medico-legal reasons; they found that in 12 cases, chronic cardiac changes were evident.

3.2 *Myocardial infarction and cerebrovascular accidents*

There have been reports of steroid users having myocardial infarctions and cerebrovascular accidents (Frankle *et al.*, 1988; Mochizuki and Richter, 1988; Ferenchick and Adelman, 1992). The cause of these cardiovascular events related to AS use are still contentious and there have been at least four hypothetical models suggested (Melchert and Welder, 1995). These include accelerated atherogenesis, induced thrombosis, vasospasm (Green *et al.*, 1993; Schror *et al.*, 1994) and direct myocardial injury (Mewis *et al.*, 1996; Nieminen *et al.*, 1996).

The first case report of myocardial infarction was in a 22-year-old AS user and was associated with markedly abnormal lipid profile with a large increase in cholesterol, but diet and genetic predisposition could not be excluded as contributing factors (McNutt *et al.*, 1988). A later report was a case in a 23-year-old AS user of 5 years who had no familial history of cardiovascular disease and was a non-smoker. He also had a deranged lipid profile that returned to normal range after discontinuing AS (Bowman *et al.*, 1989). Anabolic steroid misuse was only suspected in a sudden cardiac death in a 21-year-old after metabolites of nandrolone were discovered in the urine at post-mortem. The examination also described the presence of left ventricular hypertrophy with fibrosis but there was no evidence of atherosclerosis in the cardiac arteries (Luke *et al.*, 1990). However, other case reports implicate thrombogenic effects as the cause of myocardial infarction. A further post-mortem examination in a 22-year-old athlete showed acute thrombosis in the left main and anterior descending coronary arteries (Ferenchick, 1990).

Platelet function is one of the major constituents of the blood-clotting mechanism and one study of platelet aggregation in AS users found that there was an increased platelet sensitivity to collagen (Ferenchick and Adelman, 1992). Studies in rats show that thrombosis formation can be produced by AS suppressing prostacyclin production in arterial smooth muscle cells (Nakao *et al.*, 1981).

There has been conflicting evidence as to whether AS increases the plasma volume or increases the concentration of the haematocrit, so encouraging the development of thrombosis. Thrombosis most commonly affects the venous side of the blood system but acute ischaemic episodes affecting the arterial system cause cerebral infarction (stroke). Severe distal lower limb occlusion (Laroche, 1990) may necessitate limb amputation if embolectomy (surgical operation to remove the thrombosis) is unsuccessful or too late to be effective.

Unlike many of the adverse effects of AS, the changes to cardiovascular function continue for a long period following cessation of use (Sullivan *et al.*, 1999). A number of the deaths that have been attributed to the use of AS have occurred as a result of the negative effects of AS on the cardiovascular system. Use of AS is believed to cause changes to cellular pathology and organ physiology that are similar to those exhibited in cardiomyopathy and heart failure.

It has been debated whether use of AS is associated with increases in size of the left ventricle. Difficulties arise in validating this association because strenuous exercise has also been linked with increase in left ventricular size, and this matter is compounded because many of those that use AS participate in intense exercise activities. However, a study by Dickerman *et al.* (1998) reported that left ventricular wall thickening occurs among AS-using and non-AS-using athletes. Left ventricular wall thicknesses greater than or equal to 13 mm were considered to be higher than the 'norm' of the general population, and the study showed that all of the four elite powerlifters (non-AS users) involved in the study had thickening of the left ventricular wall at over the normal range (i.e. 13 mm or greater). Results from Dickerman *et al.*'s (1997) previous study that involved eight heavyweight competitive AS-using body-builders had shown that all of them suffered from thickening of the left ventricular wall to 13 mm or more. They concluded that AS may be indirectly responsible for this phenomenon as a result of the potential of these substances to increase strength and thereby enhance the pressor response, but left ventricular wall thickening was not restricted to AS users.

The use of other performance-enhancing and recreational drugs is prevalent among AS users (Komoroski and Rickert, 1992; Tanner *et al.*, 1995; Lenehan *et al.*, 1996); it is especially dangerous to combine any forms of illicit drugs because of the unreliability of their purity, strength and possible interactions. It is established that the majority of AS users administer their drugs without medical supervision and, in many cases, without ever having received information about AS from health care professionals or other reliable sources (Lenehan *et al.*, 1996). The use of clenbuterol in conjunction with AS has been reported to have caused a myocardial infarction in a 26-year-old male body-builder (Goldstein *et al.*, 1998). The patient was reported to have been healthy in all other respects at the time of the myocardial infarction and it is believed that AS and clenbuterol acted in synergy to result in this event.

3.3 *Blood pressure*

Most people believe that a raised blood pressure (BP) is one of the most common side-effects of AS use (Perry *et al.*, 1990a). This assumption was largely based on the results of animal experiments. The action of AS causing hypertension is still a matter of conjecture, but suggestions have been made that raised levels of 11-deoxycorticosterone may be responsible (Rockhold, 1993). Anabolic steroids inhibit the 11β-hydroxylation of 11-deoxycorticosterone to corticosterone. With this chemical pathway blocked, the amount of 11-deoxycorticosterone increases, so exerting an effect similar to excessive cortisol secretion in Cushing's syndrome.

Other suggested mechanisms include increased peripheral vascular resistance due to an enhanced reactivity to noradrenaline (Greenberg *et al.*, 1974). Steroids can increase renal secretion of renin (Katz and Roper, 1977), a hormone responsible for regulating circulatory function through the kidney and therefore having an effect on blood pressure. These hypotheses are by no means conclusive and the experimental evidence from human studies has yet to be produced.

However, the occurrence of hypertension has not been borne out by the observational studies on AS users. Most find there are no differences when monitoring blood pressure after the use of steroids (Holma, 1977a; Kleiner *et al.*, 1989). Other studies, however, have reported statistically significant increases in blood pressure with the use of AS (Freed *et al.*, 1972; Lenders *et al.*, 1988). This does not necessarily mean that this rise in blood pressure is significant clinically, as such small changes in blood pressure will have a minimal effect over a short period of time.

3.4 *Liver function*

The 17-alkylated steroids have been the type of steroid most commonly associated with detrimental effects on the liver (Hickson *et al.*, 1989). The use of some of these steroids has been withdrawn in the treatment of humans due to adverse effects but AS users still manage to obtain illicit supplies. The liver is the main organ that metabolizes steroids and clears the products into the bile (Friedl, 1993).

Nearly all studies of AS users have documented abnormalities in liver function tests with rises in alanine transaminase (ALT) (Freed *et al.*, 1975) and aspartate transaminase (AST) (Shepherd *et al.*, 1977), but some studies have found no changes in blood samples taken for liver function analysis (Hervey *et al.*, 1976). ALT and AST are also produced by muscle, heart and bone and so the interpretation of liver function assays can be difficult to analyse, as elevations in these liver enzymes can result after exercise or after tissue damage such as might be caused by injecting steroids. If the raised levels are attributable to AS then they are usually reversible after stopping steroid use or are transient even if AS use continues (Lamb, 1984). It has been suggested that future studies of AS use in athletes should monitor the enzymes lactate dehydrogenase (LDH) and alkaline phosphate (ALP), which are more specific to the function of the liver (Kibble and Ross, 1987).

Analysis of studies prior to 1984 shows that on average 46% of AS users will have abnormal liver function tests, but over 80% of these will be due to alterations in the non-specific liver enzymes ALT/AST. Abnormalities of LDH/ALP will be seen in nearly 9% of all AS users (Haupt and Rovere, 1984). Occasional reports still occur where there has been no evidence of hepatic impairment (Kuipers *et al.*, 1991).

Anabolic steroids are believed to be hepatotoxic, with oral forms of AS exhibiting higher toxicity than equivalent doses of injectable AS (Hickson *et al.*, 1989). Research by Dickerman *et al.* (1999) has questioned the level of hepatotoxicity of AS. This study measured increases in the levels of AST and ALT and two additional enzymes, gamma-glutamyltranspeptidase (GGT) and creatine kinase (CK). The subjects of the experiment included groups of body-builders using AS and body-builders not using AS. The control groups were made up of patients with viral hepatitis and non-exercising and exercising medical students. The results of the experiment showed that AST and ALT levels were elevated in the AS-using patients but elevations of GGT were not as frequent. The subjects who were suffering from hepatitis had elevated levels of GGT in addition to elevated levels of AST and ALT, the non-AS-using body-builders had elevated AST and ALT levels. Increases in ALT and AST are indicative of tissue damage but are not, in themselves, representative of damage to liver tissue. The study therefore suggests that changes in GGT levels may provide a better indication of liver abnormalities.

Cholestasis is a clinical and biochemical syndrome that results when bile flow is restricted. Anabolic steroids are recognized to cause cholestatic jaundice in patients receiving AS to treat a medical illness (Evely *et al.*, 1987). Cholestatic jaundice rarely has any fatal sequela and the adverse effects such as itching settle quickly on discontinuing the AS. There have been reports indicating that in some AS users intrahepatic cholestasis induced from AS use verged on requiring liver transplantation due to liver failure (Gurakar *et al.*, 1994).

Hepatis peliosis, a condition characterized by the formation of blood-filled sacs within the body of the liver, usually occurs in diseases such as tuberculosis. It has been associated with patients who have been prescribed AS by a physician as a treatment. In 1994 the first case was reported in a body-builder (Cabasso, 1994). Anabolic steroids are more likely to cause hyperplasia, multiple nodules or cancer (Overly *et al.*, 1984). The type of cancers associated with AS are very much dependent on the presence of the steroids and once discontinued the growth regresses (McCaughan *et al.*, 1985). This makes it questionable as to whether these tumours are, in fact, malignant. The cases in which liver tumours have proved fatal are when an unsuspected liver mass has ruptured and bled (Creagh *et al.*, 1988; Klava *et al.*, 1994).

It appears that men using AS are more prone to developing liver tumours, but they are the more benign adenomas than the primary hepatoma, which is not endocrine sensitive. Most of the androgen-associated tumours reported have been in men treated with steroids for Fanconis syndrome, an inherited form of anaemia, and as such appear to have a predisposition to this form of cancer when being treated with AS. The mechanism suggested for AS carcinogenic effect is that the steroid or one of its metabolites may be a tumour inducer. It may work as a co-factor with another compound, but its probable form of action is to promote the growth of an already existing liver tumour and encouraging the change from appearing benign to malignant (Soe *et al.*, 1992).

3.5 *Lipid profiles*

Low density lipoproteins (LDLs) deliver cholesterol from the site of synthesis in the liver to the peripheral tissues. High density lipoproteins (HDLs) reverse this mechanism, transporting cholesterol back to the liver for catabolism and excretion into the bile. HDL is, therefore, beneficial in reducing the amount of peripheral cholesterol deposition, which could cause atheroma and arteriosclerosis of the vessels of the cardiovascular circulatory system. One of the benefits of exercise is that this activity increases HDL levels, but unfortunately AS use reverses this benefit in weightlifters (Strauss *et al.*, 1982). A serum concentration of HDL below 1.0 mmol/L carries a higher risk of developing cardiovascular disease (however, specific threshold values may vary between laboratories).

Nearly all studies of HDL in AS users have documented a fall in HDL concentration (Glazer, 1991). The reduction in HDL is due to the potentiation of hepatic triglyceride lipase, a liver enzyme that regulates serum lipids (Kantor *et al.*, 1985). The 17-alkylated steroids reduce high levels more dramatically than other steroids, but the abnormalities in lipid profiles return to normal in the short term on cessation of AS use (Peterson and Fahey, 1984). Changes in lipid metabolism can remain altered for up to 5 months (Lenders *et al.*, 1988). Anabolic steroid use reduces levels of HDL by just over 50% while increasing LDL by 36%. These changes in lipid profiles may confer a threefold increase in the risk of coronary heart disease (CHD) (Cable and Todd, 1996), although genetic predispositon may have a significant role to play in some cases.

An in-depth study of two body-builders using AS showed that HDL concentrations depressed by over 69% before the fifth week of the cycle (Lajarin *et al.*, 1996). Increases of over 144% were seen in LDL and total cholesterol. These changes were reversed within 13 weeks of cessation of the steroids. It is the 17-alpha-alkylated AS that cause the most dramatic changes in adverse lipid profiles and Glazer and Suchman (1994) have shown in their study of 24 AS users administered with a 17-beta-esterified AS (nandrolone) that there were no significant changes to be found.

A study in normal male volunteers in which they were given weekly testosterone cypionate at modestly supraphysiological doses for six weeks found that there was a depression of 21% in HDL and total cholesterol/HDL ratios remained significantly elevated during testosterone administration and for four weeks after the last injection (Kouri *et al.*, 1996).

Even if lipid changes are transient, while using AS, users are exposing themselves to the premature development of peripheral vascular and coronary heart disease (Cohen *et al.*, 1986). Some AS users may be prone to cardiovascular disease due to a high cholesterol diet that some use as part of their training and nutritional scheme.

3.6 *Embolism*

The deaths of two weightlifters, both known to be AS users, have been reported to be caused by thromboembolic events (Montine and Gaede, 1992). Other cases of arterial thrombosis in young male weightlifters have also been documented (Frankle *et al.*, 1988; McNutt *et al.*, 1988; Ferenchick, 1990). Although use of AS has not been proved to be the ultimate cause of death in either of the fatalities, there are suspicions that AS abuse is associated with increased risk of thromboembolic events. Montine and Gaede (1992) report that post-mortem examination of one of these fatal cases revealed a large saddle pulmonary embolus obstructing the right and left pulmonary arteries, as well as peripheral emboli and associated infarcts. Detailed microscopic analysis showed that these emboli had developed over a period of several weeks before the terminal event.

3.7 *Hormones*

A proportion of male AS users will become infertile during the administration of steroids and this may continue for a period of months afterwards while the exogenous steroids are eliminated from the body and the newly produced sperm become mature cells. Interestingly, sexual libido may increase during this period (Moss *et al.*, 1993; Lenehan *et al.*, 1996).

Anabolic steroids inhibit the secretion of the gonadotrophin hormones, luteinizing hormone (LH) and follicle stimulating hormone (FSH), from the pituitary gland. In males LH stimulates the secretion of testosterone from the testicular interstitial cells, while FSH supports the production of sperm. Both these hormones are depressed by AS use and as a consequence reduce the sperm count (Holma, 1977b). There are also changes in the morphology of the sperm cells but this would not confer any genetic mutations or cause teratogenesis in any offspring but will simply increase the risk of infertility.

Reduction in the size of the testes in AS users has been reported (Strauss *et al.*, 1982). If the testes become too atrophied the effect may become permanent. Some AS users administer human chorionic gonadotrophin (hCG) after finishing courses of AS in the hope of accelerating the restimulation of testes to regain testicular volume and to promote spermatogenesis. Human chorionic gonadotrophin has the same action as pituitary LH, it is secreted by the placenta from pregnant women and collected from their urine.

Single doses of hCG appear to have no effect and repeated hCG treatments cause habituation of testes to natural stimulation of LH (Glass and Vigersky, 1980). The main potential side-effect of hCG administration appears to be the development of enlarged breast tissue in males (gynaecomastia) (Friedl and Yesalis, 1989). Gynaecomastia is a common occurrence and related to an increase in oestrogen levels or when androgen levels fall in comparison to the amount of oestrogen. Some AS users take an anti-oestrogen such as Tamoxifen, but this may have little effect in preventing the changes in hormonal imbalance. Oestrogen excess due to endogenous or exogenous causes results in gynaecomastia, which in AS users is due to the peripheral conversion of the androgens to oestrogen.

The earliest signs of AS-induced gynaecomastia are a laterally placed skin ridge and a circumareola halo. From the lateral side the nipple should be within the contour of the chest wall but the development of laterally placed breast tissue will cause a ridge of skin lateral to the nipple. These early signs will be lost as the breast continues to enlarge and becomes to resemble the shape of the female breast (Reyes *et al.*, 1995).

Anabolic steroid users who present with gynaecomastia but who do not declare AS use may undergo fine-needle aspiration as an aid to diagnosis (Fowler *et al.*, 1996). The resultant usual cytological findings of apocrine metaplasia in an otherwise healthy male without an adverse medication history should alert the clinician to the possibility of illicit AS use.

Extensive surgical removal of the whole tissue gives better cosmetic effects than fat suction to correct this abnormality (Aiache, 1989) as the breast tissue tends to be fibrous. There is a risk of postoperative bleeding as vascularity is highly developed.

A decrease in the ability of AS users to control the level of blood sugar has been reported (Cohen and Hickman, 1987). Their experiments showed that AS-using weightlifters have a lowered glucose tolerance and a higher production of insulin. This hormone controls serum glucose and the absence of insulin causes the condition diabetes mellitus. After a loading dose of sugar, AS users were unable to reduce the level of sugar in blood as quickly as control subjects and this was probably related to cells, which use glucose, resisting the effects and stimulation of insulin that is produced by the higher glucose levels. Reaction to levels of insulin is directly related to muscle mass and conversely muscle hypertrophy should enhance the effects of insulin.

Inability to control the levels of blood sugar efficiently may be a predictor of the development of diabetes mellitus, although this is not proven in AS users. The major problem for AS users may be the effects raised glucose levels may have on the additional risks of coronary heart disease.

3.8 *Thyroid*

The thyroid gland produces the hormones thyroxine (T4) and triiodothyronine (T3), which influence growth and metabolism of the whole body. These hormones are carried in the bloodstream by thyroxine-binding globulin (TBG). Anabolic steroids decrease the levels of T4-TBG in the blood (Alen *et al.*, 1987). One study of thyroid function in AS users found that this was still within normal limits but that there was a subclinical impairment within the function of the thyroid hormones (Deyssig and Weissel, 1993). The T4 and T3 TBG levels were reduced but thyroid-stimulating hormone and free T4 were the same as in non-AS users. The conclusion was uncertain as to whether AS may block the release or synthesis of thyroid hormones.

3.9 *Genito-urinary conditions*

There is believed to be an association between prostatic disease and AS use. Fifteen AS users were studied for changes and effects on their prostate

(Jin *et al.*, 1996). Central prostatic volume was increased by 20% and the central prostatic volume/peripheral prostatic volume ratio was increased by 77%. Serum changes showed a 47% decrease in sex hormone binding globulin, prostatic acid phosphatase was increased by 26% and LH, FSH and total testosterone were significantly reduced. Prostate specific antigen was within normal limits. This concurred with the findings in anaemic haemodialysed patients treated with nandrolone, which did not increase the prostate tumour marker (Teruel *et al.*, 1996). There may also be an association with prostatic cancer due to stimulation from excess androgens resulting from AS use (Schally and Comaru-Schally, 1987). Wemyss-Holden *et al.* (1994) researched the effects of self-administration of AS ingestion over a 15-week period in a male volunteer athlete who had a past history of routinely using AS. The results of the study showed that the athlete underwent an increase in prostatic volume, a reduction in urine flow rate, an increase in nocturnal urination, and changes in voiding patterns. The athlete was also reported to have experienced increases in libido and aggression while administering the course of AS. Although this experiment cannot provide definitive proof of an association between use of AS and prostatic changes, it does suggest that such a link exists and that there is a possibility that there may be a relationship between AS use, prostatic enlargement and bladder outflow obstruction.

A case study from Japan by Nakata (1997) reported the development of prostate cancer in an elderly man. The 81-year-old man was diagnosed with cancer of the prostate, and following questioning about his 'abnormal' hormone levels it was revealed that he had been using a medicine containing 6–9 mg of methyltestosterone, on a daily basis, for the previous 30 years. The levels of luteinizing hormone and serum testosterone were very low in the patient, and following diagnosis of prostrate cancer he was advised to stop using methyltestosterone and not to use any other androgenic substances, as such drugs can be responsible for causing these hormonal changes. There has also been one report of renal-cell carcinoma in an AS user (Bryden *et al.*, 1995).

A hypogonadal state is induced by using supraphysiological doses of AS. There is a markedly decreased natural testosterone concentration in association with testicular atrophy and impaired spermatogenesis. These conditions are produced by the negative feedback mechanism of AS on the male hypothalamic–pituitary axis and from local suppressive effects of AS on the testes. This results in hypogonadotrophic hypogonadism with a concomitant reduction in semen quality and consequent subfertility (Lloyd *et al.*, 1996).

Although thought to be reversible on discontinuation of illicit AS, there have been an increasing number of reports suggesting that low testosterone and gonadotrophin levels have persisted for over 3 years following the end of AS use. However, these AS users have been treated successfully with hCG (Turek *et al.*, 1995). Anecdotal evidence suggests that many individuals in the AS-using community self-administer hCG, a hormone obtained from the urine of pregnant women, to counteract the adverse effects that AS use induces on male sexual organs (Hart, 1993). Gill (1998) reports a case history of the successful treatment of a young male AS-using body-builder. The patient was suffering from profound hypogonadotrophic hypogonadism. Although the patient had stopped using AS he continued to suffer from the disorder. Human chorionic gonadotrophin was used to treat the patient during a course of weekly injections for a 3-month period. After treatment, the patient experienced a full recovery. It has been suggested by Gill that the medical profession should consider using hCG to treat other patients who experience hypogonadotrophic hypogonadism that has been induced by AS use. Long-term use of AS causing persistent atrophic testes may cause testicular failure secondary to fibrosis. Impotence and decreased libido can also be problematic. One case persisted for nearly a year before commencement with clomiphene to help resolve the symptomology (Bickleman *et al.*, 1995).

3.10 *Sexual behaviour*

Anabolic steroid users generally report an increased sexual drive while using AS (Lenehan *et al.*, 1996) and surveys report that more than four out of five are sexually active in the previous six months. A group of AS users and a group of non-AS-using body-builders were compared for sexual behaviour by means of a structured clinical interview. The AS users reported a significantly higher coital and orgasmic frequency but complained of erectile difficulties; however, overall the androgenic effects of the AS were to enhance sexual desire (Moss *et al.*, 1993).

There have been various reports of the transfer of HIV from and to AS users mainly from the sharing or use of contaminated injecting equipment (Sklarek *et al.*, 1984; Scott and Scott, 1989; Henrion *et al.*, 1992). Sharing behaviour may be considered the major risk factor for HIV; however, the increased sex drive reported by AS users may, if acted upon in the absence of appropriate precautions, result in the spread of sexually transmitted disease such as HIV (Lenehan and McVeigh, 1994). AS users may also have a higher number of sexual partners than the general population, which may be three times higher in AS-using males (Korkia and Stimson, 1993) with nearly two-thirds of these never using condoms with their regular partner and only 22.9% not using condoms with casual partners.

An American study found that the frequency of AS use was associated with various high-risk behaviours such as higher numbers of sexual partners in the last three months, no condom use during last intercourse and a history of sexually transmitted disease (Middleman *et al.*, 1995). The authors suggest that the behaviour in AS users should be considered as part of a risk-behaviour syndrome rather than AS use considered in isolation.

A study by Yates *et al.* (1999) investigated the psychosexual effects of three doses of testosterone cypionate in men. This research showed that each of the three doses, i.e. 100 mg, 250 mg and 500 mg weekly for a period of

14 weeks, had no effects on psychosexual function. However, one of the subjects who had received the 500 mg of testosterone cypionate developed symptoms resembling an agitated and irritable mania. This study is particularly interesting because most of the individuals that use AS, such as testosterone cypionate, administer very high doses. The conclusions of this study were that a minority of normal men may experience psychological changes if they are using doses beginning at around 500 mg per week.

Borowsky *et al.* (1997) studied the risk factors for sexual aggression among 71,594, ninth- and twelfth-grade students in the USA. Their results were based on the responses from an anonymous self-report survey, and analyses were made by comparing the responses of students reporting a history of forcing someone into a sexual act and those reporting they had never forced someone into a sexual act. It was discovered that use of AS and of other illegal drugs was associated with sexual aggression.

3.11 *Changes in metabolism*

Studies have shown that most metabolic changes during exercise are the same in AS users as in those who do not use steroids. During exercise metabolic acidosis occurs, which resolves at the same rate in both groups (McKillop *et al.*, 1989). Urea and electrolytes, such as sodium, potassium chloride and blood sugar remain within normal levels during exercise.

Serum calcium, albumin protein, phosphate and serum iron all rise temporarily during vigorous exercise. Transferrin levels remain stable and zinc and caeruloplasmin levels fall steadily. Although adrenocorticotrophic hormone (a hormone produced by the anterior lobe of the pituitary gland that stimulates the cortex of the adrenal gland) falls when AS are administered, cortisol levels are not affected (Alen *et al.*, 1985).

Studies in AS users undergoing weight training have shown that they have higher serum levels of creatine kinase (CK) (Hakkinen and Alen, 1989). Creatine kinase is an enzyme that catalyses the energy release from phosphocreatine, which is stored in muscle as a high-energy phosphate necessary for muscle contractions. Although strength training increases CK levels the effect may be increased ninefold by the concurrent use of AS (McKillop *et al.*, 1989).

3.12 *Dermatology*

Acne vulgaris is a common complication of AS use (Lamb, 1984). Large doses of AS increase the sebum excretion rate, which allows for the increased colonization of the skin by bacteria such as propionibacterium acnes

(Scott and Scott, 1992). This can cause an abnormal immunological response resulting in acne fulminans, an ulcerative and cellulitic reaction of large parts of the skin, leaving keloid scars on resolution (Heydenreich, 1989).

A case report describes acne in a 29-year-old who developed acne on his chest and back after three weeks of using nandrolone 50 mg intramuscularly twice weekly (Collins and Cotterill, 1995). Despite discontinuing the AS his skin condition deteriorated and he developed intensely inflammatory papules, pustules, nodules and pyogenic granulomata on the chest but with only minimal facial involvement. Sebum excretion was noted to have increased. He was successfully treated with cream containing clobetasol, neomycin, and nystatin with minocycline and the addition of isotretinoin at a later stage.

Local tissue reaction and allergy can occur at the site where a steroid and its base have been injected (Khankhanian *et al.*, 1992). This can produce a large tumour-like mass that would require extensive surgery if the previous history of injecting drug use was not declared. Sebaceous cysts, alopecia, hirsutism, striae atropicae, seborrheic dermatitis and furunculosis have been suggested to occur in AS users. Scars due to excessive collagen formation in the skin during tissue repair after injury with injections of AS have been documented (Scott *et al.*, 1994).

3.13 *Immunity*

Sex hormones regulate immunological function (Grossman, 1985) and are generally considered to suppress immune function, although in one study of AS users all the indices of white cell counts and lymphocyte profiles were within normal limits (Morrison, 1994). A more in-depth study has examined the immune response (Calabrese *et al.*, 1989), in which lymphocyte subpopulations, proliferation, natural killer activity and serum immunoglobulins were examined. Immunoglobulins (Ig), which are major components of the immune system, are produced by lymphocytes and plasma cells. They circulate in the blood and bind to sites on the cell walls of organisms they recognize as foreign, so helping to destroy them. IgA and IgM were the most suppressed immunoglobulins of the five classes. Testosterone suppresses cell differentiation and may enhance suppression of cell activity to cause this effect. Even though AS can suppress cell-mediated immunity in autoimmune disease, there was no significant difference in lymphocyte transformation in AS users compared to non-AS users challenged with a series of mitogens. There was also no difference in the relative distribution or number of the following lymphocytes: T cells, T-suppression/inducer cells, T-cytotoxic/suppression cells or activated T cells.

Research in mice has shown that high doses of AS have significant effects on immune responses and extrapituitary production of corticotrophin (Hughes *et al.*, 1995). Anabolic steroids applied to exercised and trained rats showed that endurance exercises as opposed to high-intensity training could correct the apparent negative effects of high doses of androgens on lymphocyte function (Ferrandez *et al.*, 1996). Nandrolone decanoate was noted to promote a redistribution of immune cells from the thymus to the spleen, impair lymphocyte mobility and the mitogen-induced proliferative response.

Doses of AS commonly used by AS-using athletes were applied to rats and were found to decrease significantly the number of neurones exhibiting cytoplasmic immunoreactivity in the rostral region of the arcuate nucleus in the brain (Menard *et al.*, 1995). Skin-test responses in rats after five days of treatment with AS showed a significant immunosuppression (Mendenhall *et al.*, 1990).

Exercise alone may affect the immune system and any changes in physiology may be wrongly attributed to AS. After endurance exercise lymphocytes are reduced in the blood and the function of natural killer cells and secretory immunity are suppressed (Pederson and Bruunsgaard, 1995). However, moderate exercise can temporarily enhance the immune system but the immunodepression of prolonged training can increase the risks of infections.

3.14 *Infections*

Anyone who injects drugs will be vulnerable to skin infections if the skin is not hygienically prepared or if injecting equipment becomes contaminated. There have been surprisingly few reports in the medical literature of abscesses or cellulitis in AS users apart from unusual presentations (Plaus and Herman, 1991). AS users should ensure they have an up-to-date tetanus vaccination.

3.14.1 ANABOLIC STEROID USE AND THE TRANSMISSION OF HIV

There are three main factors to consider when assessing the role AS may play in the transmission of HIV:

1 unprotected sex;
2 sharing injecting equipment;
3 trauma.

The two major studies of AS in the UK have indicated that a significant number of users will experience an increased libido: 60% (Lenehan *et al.*, 1996) and 50% (Korkia and Stimson, 1993). It has also been shown that 60% of steroid users never use a condom with their regular partner and 50% do not always use a condom with casual partners (Korkia and Stimson, 1993). A related issue is the use of steroids by gay men, in particular sex-trade workers.

The majority of steroid users inject: 81.3% according to Lenehan *et al.* (1996). There have been few confirmed cases of HIV infection as a direct result of AS users sharing injecting equipment or multidose vials with a couple of notable exceptions (Sklarek *et al.*, 1984; Scott and Scott, 1989). Although several studies have indicated that 'sharing' among steroid users is not a major issue in the UK, this is not the case in Canada (Melia, 1994). Of the estimated 83,000 steroid-using 11- to 18-year-olds, 29.4%, or 24,402, injected. They where then able to calculate that nearly a third of these steroid users shared injecting equipment, that is approximately 8000 11- to 18-year-olds.

A third factor is trauma, during full contact sport, or through violence. In some sports, injuries that draw blood are relatively commonplace (rugby and combat sports such as boxing and martial arts). Poor safety precautions during the treatment of these injuries can lead to cross-infection, with a subsequent risk of HIV transmission. Sporting authorities appear reluctant to address the issue: 'Whatever the rate of HIV infection, on the field transmission is certainly less frequent than hepatitis B . . . continued participation in the NFL [National Football League] of HIV infected players should remain a private decision between the player and his physician.' (Brown *et al.*, 1994). A more significant issue may be the blood-to-blood contact experienced by steroid users employed in security occupations such as nightclub doormen. Research has demonstrated the link between doormen/ bouncers and steroid use (Lenehan and McVeigh, 1996), highlighting the need for HIV prevention strategies within this section of the population.

The sharing of injecting equipment allows for the transfer of viral infections such as hepatitis B and C. The transfer of HIV by this process has already been documented in three cases (Sklarek *et al.*, 1984; Scott and Scott, 1989; Henrion *et al.*, 1992). The 1984 report described a 37-year-old man who injected AS on a weekly basis and often shared needles with his training partners, but had not done so for two years, when he developed hepatitis B. Scott and Scott (1989) reported an asymptomatic AS user who was HIV positive after sharing injecting equipment up to 60 times with a homosexual friend. It is likely that more cases will be discovered as and when AS users who have become infected and are HIV positive develop AIDS-related symptoms (Nemechek, 1991).

Research surveys in the UK confirm that AS users do share injecting equipment and at levels that are comparable to opiate- and stimulant-injecting drug users (Best and Midgley, 1999). People who have previously engaged in high-risk activities for acquiring HIV infection, such as homosexual anal intercourse and injecting drug use, also participate in body-building and inject AS (Morrison, 1994). This allows for the transfer of infections if AS users use needles and syringes or multidose vials if previously contaminated by an infected person. Lenaway *et al.* (1992) investigated a group of 33 injecting AS users. They found that seven of them (21%) reported sharing injecting equipment, while 48% had at least one sexual partner and none of these used condoms during sex, six reported that they had also injected amphetamines. In their conclusion, the authors suggested that over half of the participants were at HIV risk from unsafe injecting or sexual practice.

The potential for the spread of blood-borne infections may also be a cause for concern for the wider society. Injecting AS use has been linked with HIV, AIDS, hepatitis, mycobacterial infection and other infections in body-builders (Sklarek *et al.*, 1984; Scott and Scott, 1989; McBride *et al.*, 1996). British data suggest that there may be a danger of spreading blood-borne infections as Perry (1995) noted that 31 out of 45 new clients in a needle-exchange service in Wales admitted having shared injecting equipment. Only five respondents in the Korkia and Stimson (1993) study, which asked a very basic question on needle sharing, indicated having shared. This con-tradicts anecdotal reports from numerous needle-exchange services during the early 1990s. The danger of sharing may be substantial as a quarter of 110 interviewees said that their friends mainly injected them (Korkia and Stimson, 1993). It is also possible that AS users do not realize that, for example, drawing from a multipot vial with a needle that has already been used represents sharing. The potential problems of sharing vials and dividing drugs using syringes have been highlighted by Midgley *et al.* (2000), who interviewed 50 AS users and 40 non-users in London. They found that needle sharing was not common practice, but 19% had shared multidose vials and 17% divided drugs using syringes, both being potential routes for HIV and hepatitis infection.

'Irresponsible' sexual behaviour is a potential route for transmission of infections. Midgley *et al.* (2000) found that an increase in sex drive was more commonly reported by AS users and more AS users also engaged in sex with more than one partner, while infrequently using condoms. Similarly, Bolding *et al.* (1999) found that none of the 136 gay men who used AS had shared injecting equipment. They highlighted, however, that 21% of the AS users practised unprotected sex. The same group reported that of the total of 1004 gay men interviewed, more than 10% had injected AS and just over one-third (36%) had ever discussed this with their GP. In Merseyside, Bellis (1996) estimated that two-thirds of AS users obtained their needles from unreliable sources, such as dealers and friends. Documented infections related to AS use include: HIV, hepatitis B, mycobacterial infection, smegmatis thigh abscess and fungal infection (McBride *et al.*, 1996).

3.15 *Musculoskeletal problems*

Power athletes encounter problems of muscular injury and tendon tears or strains due to the heavy repetitive loads that are placed on these tissues during training. It is difficult to know what effect AS may have on this phenomenon above the mechanical strain load on tendons, which do not increase in size with the hypertrophy of the muscle groups. Individual case reports have included a rupture of a thumb tendon (Kramhoft and Solgaard, 1986) and muscle rupture of the triceps (Bach *et al.*, 1987). AS use may also lead to abnormal development or organization of collagen fibrils in tendons, so decreasing their tensile strength (Laseter and Russell, 1991).

Skeletal avascular necrosis has been reported to have occurred in an AS user (Pettine, 1991). This case had femoral head avascular necrosis, which can occur in those treated with glucocorticoids. This illness could require a prosthesis to replace the dead bone in the hip joint. The association between avascular necrosis and AS is unproven, but as with other side-effects of AS use it may require several years before more cases are reported. Avascular necrosis may occur during the self-administration of steroids or its effects may be delayed and occur several years after stopping AS.

Use of AS has previously been associated with increased risk of tendon rupture and musculoskeletal problems (Kramhoft and Solgaard, 1986; Bach *et al.*, 1987; Laseter and Russell, 1991). It was believed that AS were in some way capable of altering the structural properties of the tendon. However, a study by Evans *et al.* (1998) suggests that use of AS is not associated with a predisposition to tendon rupture. Evans *et al.* (1998) used electron microscopy to analyse specimens of tendon from two AS users and two non-AS users. Analysis failed to reveal any significant differences in collagen fibril structure between the two groups.

3.16 *Injecting problems*

It is important that users of injectable AS are informed about safe injecting practices and have access to clean injecting equipment. Injectable AS are intended only to be used for intramuscular injection, the safest sites for injection being the upper outer quadrant of the buttocks or the vastus lateralis. However, even if clean injecting equipment is used and users inject into either of these sites, complications may arise. Repeated injection into the same site may result in abscess formation, other complications may include damage to nerves and ligaments. Evans (1997) has reported two cases of complications resulting from use of injectable AS, where knee joint sepsis and radial nerve palsy were experienced. Other reports of abscess formation and infection with blood-borne diseases, such as HIV, have highlighted an association between AS use and 'unsafe' injecting techniques (Best and Midgley, 1999).

3.17 *Women's health*

Numerous studies have indicated that the prevalence of AS use is lower among females than males (Yesalis *et al.*, 1993b; Lenehan *et al.*, 1996;

Handelsman and Gupta, 1997; Korkia and Stimson, 1997; Lambert *et al.*, 1998). However, in recent years it has been discovered by Yesalis *et al.* (1997) that in the USA the numbers of adolescent females using AS are increasing faster than any other group.

It is generally accepted that females experience relatively greater increases in muscle strength and mass as a result of AS use than males (George, 1996a). However, anecdotal evidence circulating in underground muscle culture steroid handbooks reports tremendous strength and muscle gains from steroid use in both males and females (Duchaine, 1989; Hart, 1993). These handbooks are often written by individuals involved in the steroid-using culture and tend to contain information that is unsubstantiated by science and medicine. It is recommended by the underground steroid handbooks that female steroid users should have shorter periods of time using steroids and longer periods of abstinence than men (Duchaine, 1989).

Women may have a greater risk of developing adverse androgenic effects if they are using counterfeit or fake AS (Perry, 1995). These problems may arise because they believe that they are using an AS with low andogenicity when in fact they may be using a different AS with a higher andogenicity. Women may also experience problems if using fake or counterfeit AS because they may be using higher dosages of the substance than they realize.

Lenehan *et al.* (1996) revealed that in a sample of AS users from the north-west of England the AS-using behaviour of females was different to that of males in a number of respects. One of the most notable differences was the sources of introduction to AS. In the female-only group husbands/boyfriends/partners were the most common source of introduction to AS, but in the male group this source was not stated by any users. The male group had a higher proportion of injecting users than the female group. Females used a narrower range of AS and the numbers that used recreational or other ergogenic drugs were lower than for the males. This may be related to the fact that male AS users may take other drugs, such as Tamoxifen (nolvadex), to alleviate the AS-induced side-effects such as gynaecomastia.

Another interesting point revealed by the Lenehan *et al.* survey (1996) was that women would be less likely to continue to use AS if they became illegal to use. Research has documented the difficulty experienced by many women in admitting to use of drugs, particularly drugs such as AS that have potentially virilizing effects; this fear of exposure and its potential implications may have some influence over the responses to this question. The smaller number of females that used injectable steroids may also be related to this issue. The number of female AS users attending needle and syringe exchanges has decreased between 1992 and 1996; Awiah *et al.* (1990) have also documented a feeling of isolation from drug agencies experienced by many female injecting drug users.

Anabolic steroid use remains a predominantly male form of drug use. It is difficult to appraise the effects of AS in men and correlate them with women. Female physiology is sufficiently different that there may be more detrimental effects to their health. The research detailing side-effects in women AS users is remarkable by its scarcity. Research into women users have reported deepening in the tone of the voice, increased facial hair, enlarged clitoris, changes in sexual drive, decreased breast size, irregularities and absence of menstruation, acne, hirsuitism, alopecia and increased appetite (Strauss *et al.*, 1985; Korkia *et al.*, 1996). Although these may be conditions reported by the AS-using female, some of the effects could be attributable to intensive training. Endocrine changes that have been noted are lower levels of sex hormone-binding globulin, thyroid-binding globulins and HDL (Malarkey *et al.*, 1991).

A prospective study in using the AS nandrolone decanoate in postmenopausal women with osteoporosis found that voice virilization was expressed in a loss of high frequencies, in voice lowering and increased voice instability (Gerritsma *et al.*, 1994). Virilizing hormones in women do not cause any physical changes in the larynx but there is a shift in the production of cells of the organ from muscle to connective tissues. This causes the vocal cords to become more rigid.

Oligo/amenorrhoeic athletes have higher basal cortisol and androstenedione concentrations and have a significantly lower ratio between adrenocorticotrophic hormone (ACTH)-induced production of dehydroepiandrosterone (DHEA) and 17-alpha-hydroxyprogesterone and an increased ratio between basal androstenedione and DHEA (Lindholm *et al.*, 1995). These changes indicate that there is a redistribution of adrenal steroid metabolism towards glucocorticoid production in female endurance athletes and that hypercortisolism is a physiological change to maintain satisfactory blood glucose levels during strenuous exercise. The hypercortisolism also changes the hormone balance to a predominately catabolic state.

Those women engaging in AS use tend to be using similar doses to AS-using men (Korkia *et al.*, 1996), and for similar duration of use. It would be understandable for them to report adverse effects to the same degree as men; however, Korkia *et al.* indicated that women did not report side-effects to the same degree. This may be due to women being less likely to attend clinics for health checks and so many subclinical problems may go undetected and unnoticed.

Some women who use AS do not see the adverse effects of masculization, such as amenorrhoea, clitoromegaly or decreases in breast size, as particularly problematic. They are assumed to be acceptable effects in the perceived advantageous benefits of using AS and even increases in libido and aggression were seen as aiding performance.

3.18 *Adolescence*

The use of AS among adolescents has been increasing over the past five years. A study carried out in the United States found that young people who used

AS were more likely to use other drugs, both for recreational and for performance-enhancement purposes (Buckley *et al.*, 1988; Johnson *et al.*, 1989; Schroff, 1992). It is certain that there is pressure on this age group to conform to the ideal body images portrayed in the media. There are also concerns that the use of AS before sexual maturation may be associated with fertility problems. There are a wide variety of side-effects, physiological and psychological, associated with the use of AS by adolescents.

3.19 *Psychological effects*

Cooper *et al.* (1996) conducted a study that showed that one in three of the AS-using individuals in their research satisfied the diagnostic criteria for at least one of the personality disorders before they started to use AS. These included paranoid, schizotypal, antisocial, borderline, histrionic, narcissistic and passive–aggressive personality trait disorders. Their results also suggested that significant disturbances in personality profile are associated with, and possibly a direct result of, AS use. A study by Porcerelli and Sandler (1995) outlined a positive relationship between narcissistic personality traits and use of AS. Their study compared two groups made up of weightlifters and body-builders, one group consisting of AS users, the other of non-AS users. The AS-using group had significantly lower levels of empathy but significantly higher levels of narcissism than the non-AS-using group. The only difficulty involved in the interpretation of these results stems from the fact that personality traits prior to onset of AS use were not recorded, therefore it is impossible to conclude whether a predisposition to such traits is related to the initiation of AS use.

During the 1990s the phenomenon of road rage became a topic of significant public and media interest. The possible association between use of AS and increases in aggression and violent behaviour – 'roid rage' – have also been the focus of public attention. A study by Ellingrod *et al.* (1997) was conducted to determine the potential effects that the use of AS may have upon driving performance. Testosterone cypionate was administered to the subjects at a range of doses. The effects of 100, 250 and 500 mg per week were studied. The larger two doses are believed to be similar to the doses used by illicit AS users. The study failed to show that use of any of the doses of AS had an effect upon driving behaviour. Use of the Buss–Derkee Hostility Index also failed to show an increase in aggression in any of the six individuals involved in the study. These results were based upon driving behaviour in a semi-controlled environment and were also controlled in that certain variables that are present in non-controlled environments were eliminated from the study, for example concomitant use of other drugs, either recreational or ergogenic.

Other research by Maycock (1999) has shown that certain users of AS may experience feelings of aggression; this research also reports one case of

AS-induced 'road rage'. Another episode of aggressive driving behaviour is described in Sam Fussell's account of his own use of AS (1991). A study by Strauss *et al.* (1985) involving 10 weight-trained women AS users showed that feelings of aggressiveness were in fact perceived as being beneficial to training by six women. However, others in the study reported that problems with family members had been caused as a result of increased aggression.

There is a widely held view among the steroid-using community that certain substances are more likely to promote aggression than others (Duchaine, 1989; Hart, 1993). The testosterones and testosterone complexes (e.g. Sustanon 250 – a mixture of testosterone compounds) are regarded by many as being most often associated with feelings of aggression. This concept has not been researched and it is uncertain whether these rumours have any degree of scientific accuracy.

3.19.1 BEHAVIOURAL ASPECTS OF AS USERS

Behavioural aspects in AS users have become of interest recently and there is a concern that they may represent a public health problem. Anabolic steroids have in fact been used in the past to treat depression and some psychoses but have been superseded by the more modern pharmacotherapies. Anabolic steroids have been attributed with causing adverse psychiatric problems, which have included violence and suicides in those using AS illicitly in high doses. When used in therapeutic doses for illnesses such as anaemia and hypogonadism, psychiatric problems are rarely noted.

It is well established that there is a relationship between testosterone levels and aggressive behaviour in animals. In monkeys testosterone cypionate increased dominant behaviour in those who were dominant in the group and increased submissive responses in those who were subordinate at the start of the study (Rejeski *et al.*, 1990). In rats nandrolone decanoate reduces locomotor activity (Minkin *et al.*, 1993) and testosterone proprionate increases dominance, although copulation frequency remained unchanged (Lumia *et al.*, 1994). In female rats a combination of AS caused a decrease in activity, increased aggressiveness and eliminated some normal sexual responses (Bronson, 1996). Although recent and continuing studies support the view that AS cause behavioural changes, it remains difficult to apply these results to a human context as it is not possible to examine more sophisticated levels of emotion such as elation, depression, anger and frustration.

Testosterone enanthate has been studied for some time as an efficacious contraceptive in inducing azoospermia in normal men (WHO, 1990). These types of contraceptive studies rarely report adverse psychological reactions, and, of the small numbers that do drop out, it is only a minority of men who give psychological causes for their discontinuation from the study. Some of the problems attributed to this have been increased aggression, cyclical mood changes and increased irritability and fatigue. Testosterone replacement therapy in hypogonadal males usually decreases tiredness, irritability, anger, sadness and anxiety and can significantly improve energy levels, friendliness and feelings of well-being. However, the doses in these studies are far less than the illicit AS user would consider using and more serious consequences may be dose dependent.

Case reports published in the medical journals continue to document behavioural changes in the illicit AS user. Pope and Katz (1992) describe three men who after structured psychiatric interviews concluded that their use of AS was associated with them impulsively committing violent crimes, including murder. Dalby (1992) reports detrimental change in behaviour culminating in armed robbery after a brief exposure to AS. A five-week course of an AS caused irritability, depression and violent rages and his AS use was used as a defence in mitigation. Schulte *et al.* (1993) reported domestic violence and child abuse in a 19-year-old college football player. On discontinuation of AS, symptoms of irritability and violent outbursts resolved within two months. Several other cases of violent and criminal behaviour that may be associated with AS use, including rape and murder, have been reported, as has psychiatric illness including delusions and hallucinations (Choi and Pope, 1994; Stanley and Ward, 1994).

The first placebo-controlled prospective study of 20 volunteer men given high-dose methyltestosterone showed that AS were responsible for increases in euphoria, sexual arousal, irritability, mood swings, violent feelings, anger and hostility, distractability, confusion and forgetfulness, with one subject experiencing mania (Su *et al.*, 1993).

Survey reports have included higher numbers of AS users in their studies and have been able to investigate symptoms that would be classed as being milder adverse reactions. These would not have been severe enough to warrant case reporting on their own. Lindstrom *et al.* (1990) found that changes in mood and increased libido were the two most commonly self-reported effects of 53 male AS-using body-builders and in a questionnaire of 21 AS users attending a needle-exchange scheme it was found that they reported higher levels of alertness, irritability, anxiety, suspiciousness, negativism and aggressive attitudes towards training (a desired effect usually hoped for) and objects but not towards other people (Parrott *et al.*, 1994). Smaller numbers of AS users have been compared to controls in varying psychological tests and profiles. Choi *et al.* (1990) found that three AS users reported more self-rated aggression while using AS, which remained significantly higher than controls when off AS drugs. Perry *et al.* (1990b) found that 20 AS-using weightlifters had more somatic, depressive, anxiety, hostility and paranoid complaints when off AS drugs, and depression, anxiety and feelings of hostility were exacerbated during AS use. In 88 AS-using athletes compared to 68 non-AS users it was found that 23% experienced major mood syndromes involving mania, hypomania and major depression. Significant positive relationships were discovered between the total weekly dose of steroids used and the prevalence of mood disorders (Pope and Katz, 1994).

The small number of subjects involved in these type of studies and reliance on accurate recall of events by the subjects invite caution and critical analysis before firm conclusions can be drawn from the findings. The research material can also be confounded by AS users expecting psychological and behavioural changes due to an anticipated increase in aggression rather than a real effect and a convenient excuse for aggressive behaviour and to justify violent acts.

Blouin and Goldfield (1995) examined body image in AS users engaged in varying physical activities, and in body-builders who used AS the most, it was found that they had a significantly higher dissatisfaction with their body image with a greater drive for bulking, thinness and increased bulimic tendencies than runners and martial artists. In 20 AS users Porcerelli and Sandler (1995) found they had significantly higher scores on dimensions of pathological narcissism and lower scores for empathy on psychological profiling. Using multisource data and a cross-sectional assessment, 12 AS users were compared to a control group and it was found that although the personality traits were not different from control groups prior to AS use, subsequent use was associated with significant disturbances in personality profile on an interview schedule based on DSM-III-R [Diagnostic and Statistical Manual of Mental Disorders, 3rd edn, revised] personality disorder criteria (Cooper *et al.*, 1996).

Brower *et al.* (1991) have investigated addiction to AS in 49 weightlifters using a self-administered questionnaire. They found that at least 57% reported three or more symptoms from DSM-III-R indicating a diagnosis of dependence. Dependent users of AS used larger doses of AS, more cycles of use, had more dissatisfaction with body size and more aggressive symptoms. Statistical analysis showed that dosage and dissatisfaction with body size were the best indicators of the likelihood of the development of dependence to AS. Commencing AS use before 16 years of age, using multiple AS simultaneously and having used injectable AS were also reported to be good predictors of dependence (Brower, 1992).

An overwhelming feeling of not being big enough is a consistent predictor for a high risk of initially using AS (Brower *et al.*, 1994). Cooper (1994) has found that in a study of 12 AS-using body-builders, 10 had at least one of 11 standard personality disorders, with all of them satisfying the criteria for psychological substance abuse and nine for psychoactive substance dependence on AS. A small number of case reports reach the medical literature of dependence but these may be selected for publication for their dramatic and unusual presentation and do not allow generalizations to the populations they derive from. However, reviews of opinion on this subject continue to support the conclusion that AS result in psychological dependence and a withdrawal syndrome (Bahrke *et al.*, 1990, 1996).

Opioid-like withdrawal symptoms were induced in an AS user who felt addicted to AS and was unable to discontinue AS without experiencing withdrawal symptoms of fatigue and depression. After being given a Naloxone challenge he developed nausea, chills, dizziness, diaphoresis, piloerection and tachycardia for four hours (Tennant *et al.*, 1988). Aromatization and 5-alpha reduction are the routes of AS metabolism and produce a large number of metabolites that have varied biological effects. These compounds have a structural similarity to allopregnaolone, a neuroactive steroid that binds to membrane-bound receptors of inhibitory or excitatory neurotransmitters. These metabolities may possibly block the neuroactive steroids at the receptor level resulting in anxiety, excitability and increased aggression, or stimulate the barbiturate-like effects on the gamma-aminobutyric acid (GABA) receptors (Lukas, 1996).

Although various theories have been advanced on the mechanisms of how AS can cause addiction or dependence, they remain speculative. It is well established that corticosteroids, a related group of drugs, produce profound affective and psychiatric problems, and the megadoses of AS used by certain AS users might well induce some corticosteroid-like psychiatric effects (Pope and Katz, 1992).

In the absence of reliable studies into the mental health effects of AS, users and those providing health services for them will continue to have as the only source of information available to them the tragic reports on how individuals have claimed to be affected by their use of AS in bizarre and unusual circumstances (Williamson, 1994).

Anabolic steroid use has been associated with mood changes, antisocial, aggressive and violent behaviour and their possible role as a precursor to violent crime has been highlighted (Korkia and Stimson, 1993; Schulte *et al.*, 1993; Su *et al.*, 1993; Choi and Pope, 1994; Pope and Katz, 1994; Lenehan *et al.*, 1996; Pope *et al.*, 1996; Copeland *et al.*, 2000). These psychiatric effects appear to be similar in women (Korkia *et al.*, 1996; Gruber and Pope, 2000). AS users themselves typically describe that they feel more focused and able to train harder when they are taking AS. They also commonly describe suffering from short temper and elevated feelings of aggression. There is a strong belief among AS users that those who are 'predisposed' to verbal aggression or violent behaviour tend to act these out, while others are better able to channel heightened levels of aggression. A total of 110 interviewees were asked to estimate how they felt when taking AS, and in a separate question how they felt while not taking AS: 13% reported 'always, very often or often' urges to 'beat, injure and harm' others while on AS, while only 4% felt this way when off AS (Korkia and Stimson, 1993). Lenehan *et al.* (1996) reported that 30.6% of their sample of 386 AS users experienced urges to harm others while on AS. Currently, it is not known whether a cause-and-effect relationship exists between AS use and domestic violence and/or violent crime (Pope *et al.*, 2000), although a number of violent crimes have been associated with AS use (Dalby, 1992; Schulte *et al.*, 1993; Choi and Pope, 1994; Stanley and Ward, 1994).

In the early 1990s, the Metropolitan police reported five cases of AS-linked violent crimes, including rape and murder (Bristow, 1992). In the mid-1990s, newspapers reported on a Berkshire man who was taking AS at the time of setting fire to his house and family. Anabolic steroid use has been reported to result in accidental death, suicide and becoming a victim of a homicide (Thiblin *et al.*, 2000). Anabolic steroids may also, as part of a polydrug use syndrome, lead to accidental poisoning (Thibilin *et al.*, 2000). Thiblin *et al.* (1999) studied eight cases of suicide or suicide attempt and concluded that AS may contribute to suicide in predisposed individuals.

Prompted by a forensic evaluation of a 16-year-old boy convicted of murdering his 14-year-old girlfriend while taking AS, Pope *et al.* (2000) interviewed 133 convicts and found two cases of AS-induced crime. They concluded that AS use is an uncommon, though occasionally significant, factor in criminal behaviour. Psychiatric effects linked with AS use have consistently been shown not to be uniform across users, even with relatively high-dose administration (Brower, 1993; Su *et al.*, 1993; Pope *et al.*, 2000). The majority of the more 'naturalistic' studies, such as Korkia and Stimson (1993) and Choi *et al.* (1990) evaluating the effects of AS on mood and aggression, agree that mood changes are common and irritability and aggressive feelings are generally elevated. An interesting study with a relatively high dose of testosterone enanthate (600 mg weekly) injections did not find any differences in emotional state, mood, anger and partner perceptions before, during or after AS administration (Bhasin *et al.*, 1996). In contrast, Su *et al.* (1993) found a dose–effect relationship for both positive and negative mood, mood swings, violent feelings, anger and hostility, and cognitive symptoms with a 240-mg daily dose of methyltestosterone. Su *et al.* (1993) reported, however, that the effects were highly variable in their small ($N = 20$) sample of non-athletic men. Furthermore, they found no link between plasma androgen levels and symptoms recorded.

Williamson (1994) has speculated on the effects of expectations on the psychiatric outcomes with AS use. He points out that some users hope that AS will make them aggressive and this is what many users say themselves. On the contrary, Williamson (1994) also speculates that those who are already aggressive by nature may be more inclined to use AS; indeed, abnormal personality traits have been shown more often in AS users than in controls (Perry *et al.*, 1990b; Cooper *et al.*, 1996). To some extent, one would expect the media to pick on AS-associated violence if it was more commonplace, as they have a tendency to sensationalize issues related to AS and sporting drug use in general. The actual influence of AS on behaviour is an important issue from the public health and safety perspective; however, it is also an immensely complicated one. The sensitivity to certain AS, the interactions of heavy training, dieting, polypharmacy including psychostimulant use, black market preparations, prior personality dimensions and expectations are likely to potentiate their effects, but also make an assessment of the AS effects on mood and behaviour extremely complicated.

3.19.2 DEPENDENCY ISSUES

Anabolic steroids have already been associated with psychological addiction (Brower, 1993). There is also evidence to suggest the physiologically addictive nature of these substances (Kashkin and Kleber, 1989; Brower, 1993). There is still a degree of controversy as to whether AS can be physiologically addictive. The nature of the use of these substances, that is in cycles, has led many to believe that physiological dependence is unlikely. Studies involving the dependence of individuals using AS continuously may help to provide more information about this subject.

3.20 *Medical uses*

The use of AS for medical purposes is a relatively controversial subject. In the past the use of AS for the treatment of medical problems has decreased, this decrease has been accompanied by concern among the medial community about the potential androgenic and psychological side-effects that may result from administration of AS (Taylor, 1991; Hoberman and Yesalis, 1995). In the past AS have been used to treat hormonal abnormalities, malnutrition, burns, and for debilitating illness (Taylor, 1991; Dobs, 1999). They have also been used pre- and post-surgery for their effects of restoring a positive nitrogen balance and producing a general feeling of well-being (Wright, 1978).

In recent years, AS have been studied for their potential to be a new form of male contraceptive (WHO, 1990; Hoberman and Yesalis, 1995), and in the treatment of patients with HIV-related weight loss (Dobs, 1999; Strawford *et al.*, 1999). Anabolic steroids are believed to enhance feelings of well-being and to increase the appetite; these effects are of obvious benefit to patients suffering from HIV-related problems or AIDS itself. In addition to these effects AS are believed to promote an increase in lean muscle mass. Gains in lean muscle mass have been associated with positive effects upon the immune response system, and again this is a clear advantage in the treatment of HIV. However, one case of acute myocardial infarction suffered by a young HIV-infected patient who had been treated with AS has been reported (Varriale *et al.*, 1999). Further research is necessary to make a thorough assessment of the benefits and disadvantages of AS use for HIV-positive patients.

The AS oxandrolone has recently been used in a trial for the treatment of Duchenne muscular dystrophy. Fenichel *et al.* (1997) administered oxandrolone to 10 boys with Duchenne muscular dystrophy for a period of three months. The results of this treatment were a positive change in average muscle score in each of the boys. This compares to a predicted negative change in muscle score that might have been expected to occur after three months without oxandrolone treatment.

In a two-year randomized controlled trial, Beardsworth *et al.* (1999) in-vestigated the effects of administration of tibolone on post-menopausal bone loss at the lumbar spine and upper femur. The results from this study were encouraging, with significant differences, at all of the assessed sites, between the control group and the group administered with tibolone. However, adverse symptoms were shown to be a drawback of treatment with tibolone, some women from the tibolone-treated group withdrew from the experiment because of unacceptable side-effects, including vaginal bleeding. The number of women who found treatment with tibolone to be unacceptable was significantly smaller than the number who tolerated its effects.

3.21 *General practitioner surveys*

General practitioners (GPs) tend to be the first point of contact when medical problems arise generally, and this may be assumed to be true for AS users. Both the Department of Health study (Korkia and Stimson, 1993) and the North-West study (Lenehan *et al.*, 1996) suggest that GPs are involved in dealing with AS users. Korkia and Stimson (1993) found that 2% of their 110 interviewees had been prescribed AS by GPs, 33% had told their GP about the use of AS and 36% were receiving medical monitoring. A third of the 386 of Lenehan *et al.* (1996) interviewees had told their GP that they were taking AS, 22% (83) were receiving regular medical checks: 45 from their GP and the rest privately. Importantly, Lloyd *et al.* (1996) have raised the problem of treating subfertility in men who use AS. This can lead to lengthy, expensive, and totally unnecessary investigations unless the practitioner is made aware of drug use.

A survey of GPs in the Liverpool, Berkshire and Birmingham areas was completed by Lenehan and McVeigh (1996) to provide a more accurate picture of AS-user encounters by GPs located in different socio-economic areas. In total, of the 1224 questionnaires distributed, 520 were received giving an overall response rate of 42%: 217 (41%) were from Birmingham, 196 (38%) from Berkshire and 107 (21%) from Liverpool. Over a third (190 = 36.5%) of GPs had seen AS users in their surgeries, although only seven had seen women users. Most had seen less than three users (73%), while 30% had seen 3–5, 5% 6–11 and 1% 12–17 users in the past 12 months. Only 1% had seen large numbers (more than 18). Of the 190 GPs who had seen AS users, 103 suspected that their patients had health problems that were associated with AS use. The most commonly reported health problems were psychological and behavioural problems (21%), followed by cardiovascular (13%), dermatological (13%), musculoskeletal (9%) and liver function (7%) abnormalities, and gynaecomastia (7%). Because GPs are in a position to provide medically sound advice to AS users, questions about their confidence in providing information and advice were included. Only

4% of the respondents felt either confident or unconfident; less than a third (26%) felt quite confident; over a third (37%) felt either quite unconfident or very unconfident and the rest did not feel strongly either way. A fact worth highlighting is that in some areas GP surgeries receive separate funding for each registered drug user that is managed by the GPs either independently or through a shared care scheme with a local community drug team. AS users are not included in this category, and consequently, GPs will not receive extra funding for these patients. Time and money spent on them may be seen as non-cost-effective. Also, for ethical reasons, some GPs may be reluctant to get involved with AS users.

A similar survey was completed in Bedfordshire in 1997 (Korkia, 1997). Of the 275 questionnaires sent to GPs, 165 (60%) were returned from 18 different postal districts, including urban and rural areas. Of the respondents, 50% had seen AS users who were mainly men. The overall results of this survey were similar to those of Lenehan and McVeigh (1996). Projections from the whole sample suggest that at least 30% of Bedforshire GPs have seen AS users, depending on the experiences of the non-respondents.

Greenway and Greenway (1997) found that 18% of GPs they surveyed in West Sussex (with a response rate of 39%) had been asked to prescribe AS for non-medical reasons. Interestingly, 12% of the respondents thought that they were allowed to prescribe AS, while 17% did not know whether this was legal.

It would appear that there is a need for some training for GPs or information that they can access, with regard to prescribing AS, either in the form of leaflets or booklets or perhaps access to information via a telephone information service.

CHAPTER 4

A sporting perspective

From ancient Greece to modern-day Athens, every sportsman and woman has sought an edge over their rivals. Whether through the use of better training, improved technology or performance-enhancing substances, every competitor in the sporting arena has wanted victory. Never mind the old maxim that 'it's the taking part not the winning that matters'. The difference between fame and obscurity is what separates gold medallists from the also-rans. Drugs can often make the difference. The truth belies the myth peddled by sport's great romantics that knowledge of drug-taking among sport's elite began with Ben Johnson's expulsion from the Seoul Olympics in 1988. While he may have been the first true superstar to be banned for failing a dope test, he wasn't the first to be caught 'cheating'.

History shows how drugs have been an integral part of sport for thousands of years. More than two and a half thousand years before Johnson, ancient competitions witnessed attempts to better opponents (Csaky, 1972; Taylor, 1991).

4.1 *Performance enhancement through history*

The colourful painted tombs belonging to Egypt's rulers of more than three thousand years ago illustrate how the donkey was often sacrificed to give competitors an edge on the sports field. They would cut off the hind hooves of the ass, boil them, flavour with rose petals and swallow for what they believed to be an effective means of improving performance (Hoberman and Yesalis, 1995; Verroken, 1996).

Charnis, the Olympic two hundred metres sprint champion in 668 BC, put his prowess down to a diet of dried figs and water. His colleagues in the longer running events believed that sesame seeds would be effective by improving stamina. Some of the best Roman gladiators used strychnine and wine, and Olympians in the third century BC put their faith in mushrooms, specially cultivated for their hallucinogenic properties (Finlay and Plecket, 1976; Donohoe and Johnson, 1986). The diets of the athletes did change progressively but remained an important aspect of the training regime. Meat was believed to be an important constituent of the diet of second-century (AD) Greek athletes, and more recently, meat was also an important feature of the diet of the American Olympic team at the 1936 Olympic games held in Berlin, where beefsteak was regularly eaten by the athletes (Grivetti and Applegate, 1997).

The Vikings were renowned for fighting in a frenzied state while under the influence of vast quantities of 'magic mushrooms'. The name given to one group of raiders was used later to describe a disturbed state of mind – the Berserkers. Indian warriors in South America chewed on coca leaves as a stimulant. Such practices were commonplace (Csaky, 1972).

They did not break the rules or offend anyone's sensibilities. No word or phrase was coined to describe what people were doing, until 1889 when 'dope' first appeared in an English dictionary (Verroken, 1996). The word itself was several hundred years old before making it into print. Taken from the native 'kaffir' dialect of South Africa, 'dop' referred to a stimulating liquor, similar to brandy, made from grape skins and used in religious ceremonies by tribesmen. When it found its way into the English language it was taken to mean an opium-based mixture used to provide racehorses with extra speed and stamina.

But even by that stage, sportsmen were being caught out for drug use. The first recorded cases were of canal swimmers in Amsterdam in 1865 (Goldman, 1984). Cyclists, who have always seemed to be at the cutting edge of sport doping (Lueschen, 1993), weren't far behind in the technology of performance enhancement. In the 1870s, the most popular events on the cycle racers' calendars were those that last for 6 days, 144 hours straight of competition. Entrants would take sugar soaked in ether, nitroglycerine, caffeine, peppermint and cocaine mixtures and a cocaine–heroin combination (Voy, 1991). Deaths were inevitable. Instead of being deterred, competitors in other sports wanted to learn more about the new drug technology. Towards the end of the nineteenth century, prizefighters would consume alcohol, strychnine and other concoctions before stepping into the ring (Voy, 1991).

The Olympic games have featured a number of celebrated doping cases. The most famous of the early cases was that of runner Thomas Hicks.

Competing for the USA in the St Louis Games of 1904 he needed emergency medical treatment to revive him after winning the marathon. He had taken large amounts of strychnine, brandy and raw egg whites to help him during the race (Verroken, 1996). Four years later, Dorando Pietri was disqualified from the same event at the White City Olympics in London after receiving assistance from officials to get over the finishing line. He had collapsed after ingesting a strychnine-based potion. Even Sam Mussabini, the coach of British gold medallist sprinter Harold Abrahams, made famous in the film 'Chariots of Fire', recommended the use of strychnine for runners in the shorter track events. Perhaps the most notable death in the history of sports doping is that of the Danish cyclist Knud Jensen. He died in the 1960 Olympics held in Rome, the drugs he had taken were amphetamines and Ronicol tablets. His death is thought to have motivated the initiation of the IOC's anti-doping policies (De Merode, 1988).

Amphetamines and other stimulant drugs, such as ephedrine and strychnine, were popular in sporting communities before the discovery of AS. Amphetamine was first synthesized as a crystalline white powder in 1887, its derivative N-methamphetamine (often known as speed) was produced in 1919. It has been reported that soldiers were administered amphetamine during the Second World War to increase their alertness and delay fatigue. After the war the use of these drugs spread into society, with amphetamine abuse being popular in the 1960s for recreational and ergogenic purposes. Caffeine pills were also reported to have been used by athletes at all levels, including high school, during the 1970s (Goldman, 1984). In 1972 caffeine was removed from the IOC doping list; it has since been reintroduced as a substance illegal in concentration in the urine over 12 micrograms per millilitre.

A number of health problems, and even deaths, among the sporting community have been attributed to the use of stimulants. These substances are associated with an increased risk of myocardial infarction and heat stroke; both of these risks are exaggerated by intense physical activity, especially if this is taking place in a hot climate. As mentioned earlier, the Danish cyclist Knud Jensen died during the 1960 Rome Olympics as a result of amphetamine use. Two other members of Jensen's team also had to be admitted to hospital as a result of suspected amphetamine use (Verroken, 1996). The Tour de France of 1967 saw the death of a British cyclist called Tommy Simpson; a post-mortem proved that Simpson had used amphetamine and methamphetamine and also consumed alcohol.

In more recent times the number of elite athletes that have tested positive for amphetamines has decreased, with a higher proportion being discovered to use AS (Wallechinsky, 1996). However, use of amphetamines in professional American football has been reported to be prevalent (Goldman, 1984). Mandell (1979) researched the use of amphetamines in NFL football and discovered extensive abuse of these drugs with 60–70 mg being the average dose per man per game. He found that the reasons for amphetamine use were to increase the levels of aggression during games.

The situation in sport remains fundamentally the same today, with athletes testing positive for banned substances such as AS. The continuous development of new substances provides a wide range of choices for athletes wishing to use drugs. Advances in techniques and technologies occur in conjunction with the development of new drugs. Thus, the governing bodies of sport face an ongoing struggle to keep their tests as up to date and accurate as possible, and to develop new tests for new substances.

4.2 *Anabolic steroids*

Anabolic steroids were first developed in the 1950s, but the process that led to the manufacture of AS dates back much further. The underlying principles of AS use were common during ancient times, ingestion of animal and human tissues was a common practice for the treatment of a range of disorders. The Auyrveda of Susrata suggested that impotence could be kept at bay by eating testes (Weil, 1925; Hoberman and Yesalis, 1995), while other reports suggest that people of the Middle Ages ate testicles as an aphrodisiac. When the Pharmacopea Wirtenbergica was published in 1754, it contained lists of remedies that used horse testicles and the penises of marine mammals.

The ancient remedies persisted within society, and as the Age of Science dawned, experiments were performed to determine the scientific basis of these treatments. As the potential benefits of male hormonal extracts were being investigated, research was also undertaken to identify their active ingredients. Physiologist Charles Edouard Brown-Sequard made a significant breakthrough in 1889. Appearing before colleagues at the esteemed Societe de Biologie in Paris, he claimed to have developed a therapy to reverse the aging process (Taylor, 1991). The 72-year-old had been injecting himself for some time with extracts from the testicles of dogs and guinea pigs. Despite the faith that early pioneers, such as Brown-Sequard, had in the primitive forms of testosterone 'therapy', much of their work was disregarded by the scientific and medical communities. As a consequence, the subject remained poorly understood until many years after Brown-Sequard's experiments.

Years after these early experiments, in the 1920s, there was renewed interest in the function of the testes. McGee performed a modified version of the rooster experiment in which extract from bulls' testicles was discovered to stimulate comb growth of capons. Other research by Pezard and Caridroit and Gallagher and Koch showed similar results. The outcome of this research was that Berthold's original conclusion became accepted by the scientific community; the testes were responsible for secretion of a substance, into the bloodstream, that would restore certain 'male' characteristics in castrated animals.

Further study sought to establish more information about the chemical properties and biological functions of the substance secreted by the testes. The German scientist Adolf Butenandt managed to isolate small quantities of the androgenic hormone androsterone from 15,000 litres of urine sourced from Berlin's policemen (Butenandt and Tscherning, 1934a,b; Kochakian, 1993b). In the mid-1930s, it was demonstrated that administration of testosterone to castrated dogs (Kochakian and Murlin, 1935; Kochakian, 1935) and eunuchoid males had effects on the secondary sexual characteristics and produced a general anabolic effect. Kochakian (1976) concluded that testosterone is a general anabolic agent.

Research teams, sponsored by three rival chemical companies, tried to find more effective testosterone. Butenandt's group was funded by Schering. Another unit was backed by Organon from Holland. But it was Polish scientist Leopold Ruzicka, working for Ciba, who, in 1935, managed to beat the others and patented a process for the artificial preparation of testosterone. Both he and Butenandt shared the 1939 Nobel Chemistry Prize for their work; however, apparently influenced by the tensions of the Second World War, Butenandt declined to accept the award (Kochakian, 1993b; de Kruif, 1945). By then, commercial production of synthetic testosterone had begun.

After the hiatus caused by the war, sport began to take on board the lessons that had been learned and the potential benefits that could be harvested. The war itself had provided useful information on testosterone. It is rumoured that German soldiers heading for the front were given testosterone injections to allow them to fight harder and for longer (Wade, 1972; Wright, 1978). There is evidence that victims of the Nazi concentration camps were also prescribed the drug to build them up after the hardships of being a prisoner of war (Hoberman and Yesalis, 1995; George, 1996a).

In 1945, Paul de Kruif wrote *The Male Hormone*, a book that summarized many of the positive findings made by the chemists. According to anecdotal reports, body-builders in California began to use testosterone to help them in the gym almost immediately (Yesalis *et al.*, 1993b). However, the drug did not become an accepted part of sports practice until the 1950s. There were reports of steroid vials being found in the changing rooms used by one speed skater at the 1952 Winter Olympics in Oslo (Goldman, 1984). Four years later, the Soviet physician at the World Weightlifting Championships in Moscow told his American counterpart, Dr John Ziegler, how effective testosterone had been in guaranteeing his squad's success (Voy, 1991). Ziegler himself witnessed athletes taking the drug. He noticed how the best competitors were only visible in weightlifting circles during big meets. Ziegler decided that his own team needed to get even.

He returned home to the USA and told both the medical and sporting communities about the Soviets new 'training' regimes. He worked with Ciba on developing a drug that was as anabolic (i.e. useful in building muscle) as the preparations used in Russia but had fewer side-effects (Taylor,

1991). The result was Dianabol, or methandrostenolone. Ziegler's decision was to prove an important landmark in the spread of steroids through sport. Once more, performance enhancement for sporting purposes was difficult to distinguish from improvement for military or political gain.

After CIBA had developed Dianabol, various other pharmaceutical companies started to produce other testosterone derivatives (Taylor, 1991). In 1963, the range of available AS included Halotestin (fluoxymesterone), Adroyd (oxymetholone), Durabolin (nandrolone phenpropionate), and the steroid later used by Ben Johnson (Francis, 1990), Stanozolol (Winstrol) (Fruehan and Frawley, 1963). Despite attempts to separate the anabolic effects from the androgenic effects this has not yet been achieved.

Although research into the performance-enhancing effects of AS had slowed down in the decade of the mid-1960s to the mid-1970s, it was clear that the use of AS and other recreational and performance-enhancing drugs had increased (Goldman, 1984). The drugs that had originally been used almost exclusively in strength-dependent sports such as wrestling and body-building were becoming increasingly prevalent in other sports such as hockey, swimming, and track and field athletics (George, 1996a).

It is reported that a significant gap in credibility has existed for many years between the sporting and the scientific and medical communities. From the 1950s onwards, many of the athletes that used AS were astounded that sporting bodies could deny their positive effects on performance. In 1975, the BASM had an official policy that stated 'no known chemical agent is capable of producing both safely and effectively an improvement in performance in a healthy human subject'. This policy was published despite evidence by Freed *et al.* (1975) from their double-blind, placebo-controlled experiment that moderate doses of AS did improve the performance of weight-trained athletes. The ACSM took a similar stance on AS. President of the ACSM Dr David Lamb published an official paper suggesting that AS were merely placebos (Lamb, 1984). Again, there was evidence available at this time that suggested otherwise.

The BASM and the ACSM felt that further research on the subject of performance enhancement and AS was futile, and subsequent lack of funding for research into this area meant that there was a significant gap in research in this field for nearly a decade. However, in the 1980s a better understanding of AS, and an acceptance of accurate information, developed (Haupt and Rovere, 1984). At the 1984 conference of the ACSM it became clear to the association that their stance on AS would have to change if credibility was to be maintained (Taylor, 1991).

It is now accepted that AS do improve sporting performance providing the following three criteria are fulfilled: the athlete has been undergoing an intensive weightlifting programme before starting the course of AS, and must continue this intensive training programme throughout the course of AS; the athlete is consuming a high protein diet; and changes in the strength of the athlete are measured by the single repetition-maximal weight technique for the exercises in which the athlete trains (Haupt and Rovere, 1984). Despite rumours of out-of-competition testing for drugs, the use of AS has increased (Yesalis *et al.*, 1993a). It is now believed that elite athletes make up only a small proportion of all AS users. Use of AS for cosmetic or functional purposes is thought to be prevalent in the UK and the USA (Yesalis *et al.*, 1993b; Lenehan *et al.*, 1996). Included among these groups are individuals involved in amateur-level sport and competitive body-building (Lenehan *et al.*, 1996). It seems that regardless of the reports of harmful side-effects, individuals continue to be tempted to use AS to improve their performance, appearance, and ability to function in their occupation.

4.3 *The response of sport*

In 1967, the IOC launched a two-pronged attack on the 'cheats'. Sex tests were used for the first time at the 1967 European Athletic Championships (Todd, 1987), the first Olympic games in which they were used was in Mexico in 1968. The tests involved a medical examination and a chromosome test (Jennings, 1996). The chromosome test determines whether the athlete has the conventional female genetic make-up, i.e. two X chromosomes, as opposed to the male genetic profile of one X chromosome and one Y chromosome. The sex tests were conducted using the polymerase chain reaction (PCR), although there is a certain degree of controversy about the reliability of this method of analysis and several eminent geneticists have disputed its value (Jennings, 1996). In the 1980s, the results of Kirsten Wengler's chromosome test were such that this American swimmer was banned from women's sport. However, additional, private tests revealed that there had been vital errors in the IOC results and Wengler should not have 'failed' the chromosome test (Jennings, 1996). These tests also discriminated against women with genetic disorders that produce a genotype unlike the 'norm'.

In addition to the sex tests, the IOC also brought in a regime of drug testing. The medical committee use urine samples to test for the presence of substances that feature on the IOC banned list. If a competitor fails to give a urine sample the result shall be deemed as positive and further sanctions shall be applied to the competitor. The list of banned substances and methods has increased in length since its inception in 1968. Because of the rapid developments in technology, separate categories have had to be added to each of the doping classes named 'and related substances'. Until the addition of this category, athletes were able to use drugs that had slightly different chemical structures, but the same actions, as the drugs on the banned list.

In the early years of drug testing, athletes were usually tested after competitions. This meant that if clearance times for the drug and its metabolites were calculated correctly, then positive tests could be avoided (Verroken and

Mottram, 1996). It was also possible for athletes to use certain substances, such as AS, because the range of drugs that could be tested for was much narrower than it is today, and the sensitivity and accuracy of tests were significantly lower than today. The current IOC drug-testing procedures serve to identify athletes who have used banned substances during competition time, samples may be requested before and after an event, and it is also possible for random tests to be performed. The testing procedures are now effective in accurately detecting a range of substances, at a high level of sensitivity. However, there are shortcomings to the testing procedures. Many of the drugs that are capable of inducing improvements in performance can be used months in advance of competitions, and therefore go undetected in the tests. Strength gains resulting from the use of drugs, such as AS and human growth hormone, may be maintained after cessation of use, and provided the clearance times are calculated correctly, the user can produce a negative doping test. In short, the tests were effective for drugs, such as amphetamines, that are used immediately before an event, but they were unable to reveal the use of drugs in the period leading up to competition time (Dubin, 1990).

Improvements in technology, and alterations in testing procedures, theoretically mean that drug-using athletes have a higher chance of detection. But even in the early stages of doping control, methods to avoid detection in tests have been used. It seems that developments in testing procedures are matched, or in some cases outrun, by improvements in technologies to avoid detection. Simple methods of detection avoidance, such as substitution of urine samples, have progressed to more complex technologies such as the use of masking agents.

Techniques to avoid detection are acknowledged to have been perfected by certain coaches and team doctors (Goldman, 1984; Voy, 1991). Masking agents, substances with the ability to hide the use of banned drugs, are just one example of the methods used. Some are simple diuretics, used to reduce the concentration of drugs in urine to make detection more difficult. Others are even more simple, including the use of lemon juice and vinegar.

Athletes have also been reported to have used condoms filled with clean urine, and catheterization methods whereby other people's steroid-free urine is inserted into their bladders (Verroken, 1996). More elaborate methods of beating the test have surfaced. One popular compound was called Defend. Marketed by an American company, its virtues were extolled in a nationwide advertising campaign that claimed it was able to 'eliminate the detection of metabolites (the by-products of steroids) in your urine that could trigger a positive test result'. Urine that is freeze-dried has also become popular in the USA: mix with warm water and the manufacturers claim that a person keen to beat the test will have a guaranteed steroid-free urine sample to help them do it. The biggest demand for this product came not from athletes but from workers in America, where urine tests for alcohol and recreational drugs are routine.

The 1976 Olympics proved to be the first real test for Professor Raymond Brook's steroids analysis. There had already been one catch in international competition. Dutch decathlete Eduard de Noorlander had gained the dubious distinction of being the first athlete ever to be disqualified after failing a steroids test. In Montreal, eight athletes failed.

Four years later, in the Moscow Olympics of 1980, no positives were reported and the Games were seen as a showpiece for Leonid Brezhnev's Communist regime. In Los Angeles in 1984, there were 11 steroid positives. A further nine positives were recorded by analysts. Nothing was ever done about these 'missing' positives. The scandal did not come to light for some time. It became clear that even if the IOC had really wanted to impose penalties on the guilty parties, they couldn't. The documents containing the identities of the athletes who had failed the tests had been shredded (Jennings, 1996).

The Los Angeles fiasco was thrown into a new light when considered in the context of two things that had happened in the previous 12 months. In 1983, athletes gathered in Caracas for the Pan-American Games. Fifteen athletes from 10 countries (including the USA and Canada) were disqualified after testing positive for steroids. They had been caught out by the introduction of more sensitive equipment – the gas chromotography–mass spectrometry machine – by the competition's organizers. In addition to the penalized athletes (who between them had won a total of 23 medals), 34 other American athletes had departed suddenly for home without competing.

In 1988 in Seoul, there were three steroid positives. Ben Johnson was, at the time of his positive test, the biggest athlete in the world. His exploits in the 100 metres had eclipsed those of Carl Lewis, the four-times champion in Los Angeles. In Rome's Athletic World Championships in 1987, he had beaten Calvin Smith's time of 9.93 seconds for the event to become the fastest man on the planet. In Seoul he reduced this to an incredible 9.79 seconds. However, he gave a urine sample that proved positive for Stanozolol.

The Canadian government ordered hearings into allegations that Ben Johnson was not the only Canadian athlete to have used steroids. The inquiry was chaired by Judge Charles Dubin. Johnson and many sportspeople involved in athletics and weightlifting admitted their steroid use. Similar commissions of inquiry in Australia and the United States uncovered similar testimonies.

There were no positives for AS at the 1992 Games in Barcelona but perhaps that wasn't too much of a shock. While drug testers had been able to work out how to trace steroids, athletes had simply moved onto substances that were then, and some still are, undetectable.

In response to the continually changing challenge posed by the doping athlete, the sports community has produced a list of banned drugs. The list is overseen ultimately by the IOC although slight variations from it exist in various sports and various countries. Doping, states the IOC, is the 'administration of or use by a competing athlete of any substance foreign to the body or any physiological substance taken in abnormal quantity or taken by an abnormal route into the body with the sole intention of increasing in an artificial and unfair manner his or her performance in competition'.

The list divides the banned drugs into categories:

Stimulants, including amphetamine and ephedrine;
Narcotic analgesics (painkillers), including codeine and morphine;
Anabolic agents, including anabolic steroids;
Diuretics (used as slimming aids and masking agents);
Peptide hormones, including Human Growth Hormone;
Agents with anti-oestrogenic properties such as tamoxifen;
Masking agents such as probenicid;
Pharmacological, chemical and physical manipulation, gene doping and the enhancement of oxygen transfer;
Drugs subject to restrictions include cannabis and betablockers.

Among the difficulties faced by the IOC in introducing doping policies is the problem of defining doping. There is a huge range of opportunities available through which athletes can improve their performance. Use of sophisticated equipment has improved the world records for a number of events, including high jump and cycling (Williams, 1997). Athletes from countries where the financial burden of sport is a great strain on the economy may face a disadvantage in that their competitors may have access to superior equipment and training facilities. It could be argued that this situation is unfair and that there should not be a differentiation between use of any artificial means of performance enhancement.

It is also interesting that certain substances that have been associated with performance enhancement are not placed on the banned list. Consequently athletes are using these drugs before their use might be banned. At present, creatine is not on the IOC list of prohibited substances. A number of studies have associated increases in strength with the use of creatine (Williams and Brach, 1998). Unlike many of the other prohibited substances, creatine may be purchased as an over-the-counter food supplement. It would therefore be difficult for sporting bodies to attempt to successfully control the use of this substance. It has also been suggested that creatine-using athletes may maintain any gains in strength for up to three weeks after cessation of use (Brodie and Towse, 1999). It is unclear whether creatine will eventually be placed on the IOC's list of banned substances.

Other substances have fallen under similar analysis. It has been debated whether females using the contraceptive pill experience ergogenic effects (Goldman, 1984), and the performance-enhancing effects of androstenedione and dietary boron are also under investigation. Dietary supplements of boron have been suggested by Naghii (1999) to elevate the levels of endogenous steroid hormones. Androstenedione is on the IOC banned list, but it is perfectly legal for this substance to be used in sports such as baseball. This drug has been the subject of controversy in American baseball, and Mark McGwire's use of this substance was exposed in 1998. Androstenedione is believed to have anabolic properties and acts by raising the levels of testosterone (Wilstein, 1998).

4.4 *Eastern European doping 'regimes'*

Reliable sources have exposed the doping programmes that existed in East Germany (Hoberman, 1990). The doping of athletes in East Germany was backed by state-funded research into ergogenic drugs and methods to avoid their detection (Dickman, 1991). The research involved a number of the East German scientific and sports institutions and the state-owned pharmaceutical organization Jenapharm. It has been estimated that up to 1500 individuals from the scientific, medical and sporting communities worked on the plan. The exposure of this plan occurred after 20 East German swim coaches admitted they had administered world-class swimmers with AS throughout the 1970s and 1980s (Noden, 1994). Kornelia Ender, a successful East German swimmer, stated that, while she was in training, her coaches had administered injections which they told her would help post-competition recuperation. She believes these injections were linked with a gain in muscle mass of 18 pounds.

Athletes in Eastern Bloc countries were not just exposed to AS (Goldman, 1984). There are also rumours that young female gymnasts were given drugs to halt their growth process. Synthetic forms of the natural hormone progesterone, e.g. medroxyprogesterone acetate, are believed to delay the onset of puberty by suppressing ovulation and thus menstruation; this is sometimes called a 'brake' drug. Doping programmes are also believed to have existed in other former Soviet Bloc countries as well as in the former Soviet Union itself (Hoberman, 1990).

4.5 *Tour de France 1998*

The 1998 Tour de France created one of the biggest sport scandals of the twentieth century. Cycling has often been identified as being at the forefront of the use of drugs in sport. Prior to the establishment of the Tour in 1903, the six-day bicycle races of the 1890s were considered to be the beginning of modern doping. Riders' coffee was 'boosted' with extra caffeine and peppermint, and as the race progressed the mixture was spiked with increasing doses of cocaine and strychnine, brandy was also frequently added. The Tour of 1998 confirmed many of the suspicions that drug use remained part of the subculture of long-distance cycling. While the Festina team were originally implicated in the scandal, suspicion soon fell on all competitors from all teams.

The problem for Festina began when the team masseur Willy Voet was stopped at the French/Belgium border where it was discovered he was carrying AS and ampoules of erythropoeitin (EPO). Initially, Festina and the riders denied all knowledge of Voet's drug cache. The team leader, cyclist Richard Virenque, denied using the drugs himself but admitted that drug use was common in the team, although he was later to admit using drugs himself. He claimed that organized distribution of drugs was common practice in all of the teams competing in the Tour. The TVM team had EPO found in one of its official cars and its riders were forced to give blood, urine and hair samples. The other riders of the Tour carried out two 'strikes' and refused to ride. The TVM team withdrew from the Tour followed by four others, while the Festina team was disqualified.

Perhaps this event provides a very clear example not only of individuals using drugs in a sporting context but also of the systematic distribution of drugs to athletes organized by team officials and doctors. It is difficult to imagine that organizers of the Tour and similar races were ignorant of the drug use which it transpires has been a part of the Tour since its inception. Organizers and officials have at best 'turned a blind eye' and at worst colluded with the cyclists in their doping regimes. The repercussions of the '98 Tour are likely to be felt for some time to come.

4.6 *Nandrolone*

A number of sportsmen and women have tested positive in the past few years for the AS nandrolone, many of whom have denied any wrongdoing. Linford Christie, the British sprinter and coach, became the most high-profile culprit after the IAAF, the governing body of world athletics, imposed a two-year ban on him for testing positive for nandrolone. Similar bans were given to sprinter Dougie Walker and Britain's former number-one 400-metre hurdler, Gary Cadogan, all for nandrolone offences. All protested their innocence.

Evidence, based on research carried out at Aberdeen University, claims that nandrolone might be produced naturally by the body through a combination of athletes taking dietary supplements and training vigorously. There are many other sportsmen from around the world who have also tested positive for nandrolone. French footballer Christophe Dugarry, Spencer Smith, Britain's former world triathlon champion, and Merlene Ottey, the Jamaican sprinter, have also tested positive but say they are innocent. Petr Korda, the Czech tennis player, was banned from playing professional tennis for two years, although he was later cleared on appeal.

The sports world appears to be split between those who claim that there could be natural reasons for the high number of positive nandrolone tests and those who argue that it underlines the rise of cheating through drug use. Professor Ron Maughan carried out research into nandrolone, and found that when athletes exercised without taking supplements, nandrolone levels were below two nanograms, the legal limit, but when they exercised while taking dietary supplements they tested positive.

UK Sport, the organization responsible for carrying out drug tests on athletes in the UK, stated that there was a 65% increase in positive tests for AS from 20 in 1998–9 to 33 in 1999–2000, and three-quarters of the positive tests were for nandrolone. But a committee set up by UK Sport to investigate nandrolone concluded that many of the health supplements that have recently flooded the market could be to blame.

Italy's National Federation cleared two athletes of deliberately taking nandrolone after they proved their nutritional supplements had been spiked. It is the first time any athlete has been acquitted after establishing a link between a positive test and a supplement. Giuliano Battocletti, Italy's half-marathon champion, and Ilaria Sighele, a young woman sprinter, each tested positive for nandrolone. Analysis on the remainder of the nutritional product that both had been using showed it contained nandrolone.

In Germany a junior javelin thrower, Carolin Soboll, and third-division footballer, Manuel Cornelius of Borussia Berlin, escaped bans after it was discovered that the US-manufactured creatine supplement they had been taking also contained nandrolone. But the IOC's stance confirms that it will maintain its policy of strict liability, which means that athletes are wholly responsible for what they ingest. An instance of their committment to this policy can be seen in the case of the young Romanian gymnast Raducan who was stripped of her gold medal at the Sydney Olympics, 2000, after testing positive for the stimulant ephedrine, contained in a cold remedy prescribed by the team doctor.

The IOC has now warned athletes to avoid taking nutritional supplements.

4.7 *Doping outside of the Olympics*

Outside of the Olympics and track and field athletics, many sportsmen and women have been caught for taking steroids. One such sportsman, the South African rugby league player Jamie Bloem, had claimed drug-taking was 'rife' – a comment that earned him a severe rebuke from Rugby League officials. The South African rugby union team were described as the 'undisputed steroid kings of rugby' (Walsh, 1998). Between 1992 and 1998, eight senior players tested positive for various AS. Italian football has been reported to have a serious doping problem. The coach of the Roma football team, Zeman, stated that 'Performance-enhancing drugs are widely used in the league'. Thomas Doll, who formerly played for the Italian team Bari, tested positive for the steroid benzbromarone in March 1998 (Walsh, 1998).

In American football steroid use has in the past been acknowledged as common. In his 1994 book *You're Okay, it's Just a Bruise*, team physician Robert Huizenga (1994) detailed some of the drug habits of the Los Angeles (Oakland) Raiders. There are also reports that coaches would turn a blind eye to this type of drug abuse (Goldman, 1984). Players could be dropped by teams for alcohol abuse but not for using steroids. Huizenga, perhaps best known in the US as OJ Simpson's personal doctor, has also experienced use of steroids by players in ice hockey, cyclists and boxers. In 1996, the first jockey to be caught using steroids was banned. Use of amphetamines and cocaine has also been seen in American football at the professional, collegiate and high-school levels (Wadler and Hainline, 1989). The cocaine-related deaths of professional footballer Don Rogers and professional basketball player Len Bias both served to raise public awareness of the use of this drug in the sporting community. Both athletes are believed to have suffered from myocardial infarction (Cantwell and Rose, 1986).

4.8 *The future*

More recent technological advances have brought an increasing number of athletes testing positive for synthetically produced hormones, such as genetically engineered human growth hormone (hGH), and products such as EPO, a means of blood doping (Armstrong and Reilly, 1996; George, 1996a).

The use of growth hormone by athletes in the 1990s is associated with the production of genetically engineered hGH. Before the advent of genetic engineering this hormone was taken from the pituitary glands of cadavers, it was mainly used in the treatment of short stature in children; however, the development of Creutzfeldt–Jakob disease in several patients who had been treated with this drug led to a reduction in its use in medicine and athletics (Wadler and Hainline, 1989). Evidence now suggests that hGH (Somatropin), a genetically engineered form of the hormone, is being used by athletes for its anabolic properties. There are also reports that certain parents are administering their children with this drug with the hope of making them grow tall enough to be successful in sports such as basketball. Research into the potential effects of the use of hGH has shown that it is associated with acromegaly and complications resulting from excessive growth of internal organs, such as the heart.

Erythropoietin is used to raise the red blood cell count and thereby increase the athlete's ability to transport oxygen around the body. It has been the subject of the recent (1998) Tour de France doping scandal, in which the Festina team were linked with the use of this drug. Alex Zulle, one of the riders to be suspended from the race as a result of EPO use, said 'I took it because I had to, in order to stay competitive. It's the same as when everybody is breaking the speed limit on the motorway, but I'm the one who got caught' (Whittle, 1998). Cross-country skiing and cycling have adopted the stance of testing the haematocrit levels of athletes and preventing them from competing if the haematocrit levels are above 50%. While the authorities cannot state that athletes above this limit are using a drug such as EPO to elevate their red blood cell count, they are able to prevent them competing on the grounds that to compete would be a risk to their health.

A new form of 'cheating' that advances in technology could make a reality in the not too distant future is genetic engineering. This could result in athletes being 'created' with all the attributes to be successful in a particular sport. This might be by ensuring their height, muscularity, speed or endurance is maximized to facilitate success in sport. What once might have been considered science fiction now rests firmly within a biotechnological reality. How sport should respond to this is the matter for much debate among the administrators of sport.

4.9 *The IOC prohibited substance list*

Anabolic steroids are only one type of performance-enhancing drugs. Many others exist and many of these drugs that were initially used by athletes for performance enhancement are now used by individuals whose aim is to improve their physique for cosmetic reasons. The IOC's prohibited substance list provides a useful framework to discuss some of these drugs. This list is that employed by the IOC. In future the role of updating and reviewing the list will become the remit of the World Anti-Doping Agency (WADA) which is discussed in section 4.10. Any changes to the list are published on the IOC and WADA websites.

PART I. PROHIBITED CLASSES OF SUBSTANCES

A number of classes of drugs have been banned by the IOC. These include:

1.A Stimulants
1.B Narcotics
1.C Anabolic agents
1.D Diuretics
1.E Peptide hormones, mimetics and analogues
1.F Agents with anti-oestrogenic activity
1.G Masking agents

A subgroup called 'and related substances' has been added to each of the categories above, as a result of the development of certain drugs with similar chemical structures and actions to those mentioned above.

1.A. Stimulants

Stimulants have been clinically proven to be associated with an increase in competitiveness (Voy, 1991). Although the drugs mentioned below may have positive effects upon sporting performance, they are also associated with specific adverse symptoms and may have the potential to become psychologically or physically addictive.

Prohibited classes of substances in this category include:

amineptine, amiphenazole, amphetamines, bromantan, caffeine, carphedon, cocaine, ephedrines, fencamfamine, mesocarb, pentetrazol, pipradol, salbutamol, salmeterol, terbutaline, and related substances.

Special rules surround a number of these stimulants. For a sportsman to have a positive test for caffeine, the concentration of caffeine in the urine must be greater than 12 micrograms per millilitre. Caffeine is present in tea and coffee and certain soft drinks, it is also used as an ingredient in many cold remedies and painkillers; this rule makes it possible for contestants to consume moderate amounts of these products without testing positive.

Ephedrine, cathine and methylephedrine are also under certain restrictions. The definition of a positive test for these drugs is a concentration in urine greater than 5 micrograms per millilitre. For phenylpropanolamine and pseudoephedrine, a concentration in urine greater than 10 micrograms per millilitre is defined as positive. If more than one of these substances has been used by a contestant, a sum of the respective concentrations greater than 10 micrograms per millilitre shall be defined as positive.

Salbutamol and terbutaline are permitted if the contestant has provided written notification of asthma and/or exercise-induced asthma from a respiratory or team physician. Contestants suffering from these conditions may only use these drugs via an inhaler.

It should also be noted that all imidazole preparations can be used in topical preparations, phenylephrine is also permitted if used in topical preparations (e.g. nasal or ophthalmological). Vasoconstrictors, such as adrenaline, may be administered with local anaesthetic agents.

Amphetamines

Amphetamine was first synthesized in 1920. It has been used for a variety of therapeutic purposes over the years, including the treatment of narcolepsy, depression, anxiety, and hyperactivity in children. The therapeutic use of amphetamine has been significantly reduced in Britain and the USA since evidence was found for its adverse symptoms and the potential for psychological addiction (George, 1996b). The main uses of amphetamine in medicine are for the treatment of attention deficit disorder, childhood hyperkinetic syndrome, and somnolence in certain nervous system diseases (Wadler and Hainline, 1989).

Amphetamines are thought to have a number of pharmacological effects, including increasing the liberation of endogenous catecholamines, displacement of catecholamines from binding sites, inhibition of enzymes of metabolism (e.g. monoamine oxidase), interference with reuptake, and action as a false transmitter (Lombardo, 1986).

Evidence suggests that the use of amphetamines can be associated with enhancement of speed, power, endurance, concentration, and fine motor coordination. These factors all have roles in sporting performance so it is unsurprising that these drugs have been used by athletes. A review by Weiss and Laties (1962) noted that amphetamine use does improve performance in a variety of tasks and this is not the result of the normalization of fatigue responses. The tasks examined by Weiss and Laties included (a) work output by subjects on a bicycle ergometer, (b) performance on military exercises, and (c) performance during flying or driving missions.

Despite the positive effects of their use, these drugs are associated with a wide range of adverse symptoms. The adverse symptoms may be experienced by chronic or 'first-time' users (Wadler and Hainline, 1989).

Many of the adverse effects of amphetamine abuse are behavioural. These symptoms are dose dependent and are thought to result from the stimulation of dopamine and noradrenaline receptors (George, 1996b). The symptoms include restlessness, dizziness, tremor, irritability and insomnia, and these effects are more common when high doses of amphetamine are used (Weiner, 1985). Chronic abuse of amphetamines may result in compulsive and stereotypic repetitive behaviour, or the development of psychotic delusions and paranoia (Langston and Langston, 1986; Fischman, 1987).

Other effects that have been associated with misuse of amphetamines are more severe and can involve physical or permanent neurological changes. Effects such as hypertension, angina and arrhythmia have been shown to be caused by amphetamine abuse (Weiner, 1985; Guyton, 1986). Amphetamines limit the cooling of blood and hence increase the risk of heatstroke, this effect occurs because the drugs cause a redistribution of the blood away from the skin. The effects of exercise, particularly in hot climates, in addition to this effect have led to the deaths of the two cyclists Jenson and Simpson (George, 1996b).

Although there is evidence that the use of amphetamine does improve certain aspects of sporting performance, other studies have shown that these effects may be outweighed by the adverse effects mentioned earlier (George, 1996b).

Caffeine

Caffeine is probably one of the most frequently used stimulants in the world. It is found in drinks of tea and coffee and many soft drinks. Caffeine may also be present in cold and flu remedies and painkillers. Despite being accepted by society and having wide-scale availability, caffeine is a potent and potentially addictive drug (Wadler and Hainline, 1989). Its use has been associated with a number of adverse effects including tremors, anxiety, cramps and headaches (George, 1996b). Although moderate doses of caffeine are permitted by the IOC, consumption of approximately six cups of coffee two hours before a test could lead to a positive result (Work, 1991). Caffeine inhibits the enzyme phosphodiesterase and has an antagonistic effect at central adenosine receptors.

The effects of caffeine include increased gastric acid and pepsin secretion, and also increased secretion into the small intestine; increased heart rate, stroke volume, cardiac output and blood pressure at rest; tachycardia; increased lipolysis; increased contractility of skeletal muscles; increased oxygen consumption and metabolic rate; increased diuresis; increased anti-nociceptive action of non-steroidal anti-inflammatory drugs (NSAIDs), and it exerts a mild anti-nociceptive action itself (George, 1996b).

Research by Bellet *et al.* (1965) suggested that caffeine may enhance the utilization of fats, hence sparing glycogen stores. This overall effect could better the endurance of athletes. There are a number of other reasons why caffeine has been used to enhance athletic performance. Intake of caffeine may significantly increase the muscle tension in the adductor pollicis muscle, this increase was observed in both fatigued and non-fatigued subjects (Lopes *et al.*, 1983). Use of caffeine has also been associated with an increase in alertness and a decreased perception of fatigue (Lombardo, 1986). Although these effects may enhance performance in endurance activities, caffeine does not significantly improve performance in intense, short-term activities (Van Handel, 1980).

Cocaine

Cocaine use has been well documented over the years but a number of its exact effects are still unclear (George, 1996b). It is associated with a variety of side-effects and is highly addictive, the incidence of sudden death increases with the increased use of cocaine (Duda, 1986a; Ring and Butman, 1986; Weiss, 1986). The deaths of professional basketball player Len Bias and professional American football player Don Rogers in 1986 were both linked with cocaine abuse, it is believed that they both suffered from a myocardial infarction (Cantwell and Rose, 1986). Awareness of the relevance of this drug in the sporting community was thought to be raised by these deaths.

Although cocaine has a shorter duration of action than amphetamine, both have similar effects upon mood states. Enhancements of friendliness, arousal, elation, vigour, and positive mood state are common to use of these two drugs (Fischman, 1987). They also have moderately similar effects upon the brain. The concentrations of dopaminergic and noradrenergic transmitters at the neuronal synapses are increased by cocaine and amphetamines. However, cocaine blocks the reuptake of dopamine whereas amphetamine enhances release of dopamine and then blocks its reuptake (Nunes and Rosecan, 1987).

Research has shown that the effects of cocaine use may be due to the reinforcing circuitry of the mesocortical and mesolimbic dopamine tracts. The self re-exciting nature of this circuitry enhances the reward or 'pleasure', and can influence the user to crave the drug (Miller *et al.*, 1987). If cocaine is used repetitively the effects upon behaviour are exaggerated, tolerance to the subjective effects of the drug occurs but the reinforcing effects remain (Fischman, 1987).

A chronic symptom of cocaine use is epileptogenesis (George, 1996b). Epileptogenesis is the stimulation of epileptic seizures, and this effect was first reported to be associated with cocaine use in 1922 (Myers and Earnest, 1984; Wadler and Hainline, 1989). The effect increases with increase in frequency of cocaine use. A range of other adverse effects may occur as a result of cocaine misuse, including cardiac arrhythmias, cerebrovascular accidents (strokes), myocardial infarction, rhabdomyolisis (disease characterized by destruction of skeletal muscle) with renal and hepatic failure, and hyperpyrexia (elevation of body temperature above 106°F) (George, 1996b). Intense athletic activity in conjunction with the use of cocaine may further increase the potential for cardiovascular problems, such as myocardial infarction and cardiac arrhythmias.

A review by Conlee (1991) stated that all of the studies carried out before 1983 relating to the performance-enhancing qualities of cocaine abuse were contradictory and scientifically inaccurate. However, George (1996b) reviewed the studies of cocaine abuse and reported that cocaine did not improve running times within a dose range of 0.1–20.0 mg/kg body weight, and at doses of 12.5 mg/kg body weight running times were in fact inferior. As yet, there is no explanation as to why cocaine may reduce endurance.

Ephedrines

These drugs are central nervous system stimulants. In the past, users have combined these types of drugs with caffeine to produce an effect similar to that produced by amphetamines. They are ingredients in many over-the-counter medicines, such as cold and flu remedies, and painkillers. The action of ephedrine displaces norepinephrine and other monoamine transmitters from storage sites (Lake and Quirk, 1984). This action is enhanced by intraneuronal monoamine oxidase resistance (Weiner, 1985). Ephedrines also have effects on alpha and beta receptors and are associated with alpha adrenergic activity (Pentel, 1984).

Ephedrine has a similar chemical structure to amphetamine and the psychological effects of the two types of drugs are alike. Ephedrine tends to exert milder effects than similar doses of amphetamine, but, at high doses, euphoria and increased alertness may be observed. Other effects that are associated with the misuse of ephedrines include increased pulse rate, elevated blood pressure, bronchodilation and behavioural changes such as psychosis, hallucinations and compulsive behaviour (Wadler and Hainline, 1989).

There is no conclusive evidence for improvement in sporting performance following use of ephedrines. Lombardo (1986) suggests that the intense levels of anxiety and the increased awareness of heart action may be the two main reasons why the use of ephedrine in sports is not as prevalent as the use of other stimulants.

1.B. Narcotics

Traditionally narcotics have been used to relieve pain; however, they are widely used for recreational purposes (Verroken, 1996). Narcotics are thought to give athletes a higher threshold of pain and a sudden rush of euphoria (Voy, 1991). Serious risks are associated with the use of narcotics, they are highly addictive, both psychologically and physically, and can cause respiratory depression. Suggestions have been made that narcotics may be used in the sporting community to relieve competition nerves and to aid relaxation (Anderson and McKeag, 1985).

The following narcotics have been banned by the IOC:

> buprenorphine, dextromoramide, diamorphine (heroin), methadone, morphine, pentazocine, pethidine, and related substances.

Opiates act upon the opioid receptors of the central nervous system and the gastrointestinal tract (Jaffe, 1985). Specific receptors are targeted by different narcotics, and the effects exerted by these reactions may vary. For example; morphine targets mu2 receptors and produces the effects of respiratory depression and dopamine turnover in the brain whereas heroin targets mu1 and stimulates acetylcholine turnover in the brain (Pasternak, 1982).

Major adverse effects linked with the misuse of narcotics include nausea, vomiting, dizziness, dysphoria, pruritus (severe itching), constipation and delirium (Khantzian and McKenna, 1979; Gold and Estroff, 1984; Jaffe and Martin, 1985). Withdrawal from narcotics is also associated with a number of symptoms. Users experience cravings, restlessness, nausea, vomiting, diarrhoea, muscle cramps/spasms, generalized central nervous system hyperexcitability and potential cardiovascular collapse.

There have been no studies to show that misuse of narcotics adversely affects sporting performance. Studies of chronic narcotic users and age-matched controls have shown that there is no significant difference between the two groups with regard to motor strength, rapid alternating movements, eye–hand coordination, visual perception and cognitive skills (Bruhn and Maage, 1975). The indirect effects of narcotics upon sporting performance may be related to the fact that athletes using narcotics to mask injuries may be putting their long-term health at risk. Training while suffering from an injury may worsen the condition and hence make it more difficult for the athlete to make a fast and complete recovery.

1.C. Anabolic agents

Anabolic-androgenic steroids

Anabolic steroids are synthetic derivatives of testosterone. They were first developed in the early 1930s and since then significant efforts have been made to dissociate the anabolic effects from the androgenic effects (Haupt and Rovere, 1984). Reports of AS use among the sporting community have been numerous. The positive drugs test of the sprinter Ben Johnson is perhaps the most memorable case of steroid misuse. Johnson tested positive for the AS stanozolol following his gold medal winning performance at the Olympic games of 1988.

Anabolic-androgenic steroids banned by the IOC include:

> clostebol, fluoxymesterone, methandienone, metenolone, nandrolone, 19-norandrostenediol, 19-norandrostendione, oxandrolone, stanozolol, and related substances
> androstenediol, androstenedione, dehydroepiandrosterone (DHEA), dihydrotestosterone, testosterone, and related substances

The IOC states that 'evidence obtained from metabolic profiles and/or isotopic ratio measurements may be used to draw definitive conclusions'.

If the urine sample of a competitor has a testosterone to epitestosterone ratio greater than 6 to 1 the sample shall be defined as positive. Evidence of a medical condition, such as low epitestosterone excretion, androgen-producing tumour, or enzyme deficiencies, is the only accepted reason for a positive test. If an athlete has tested positive for these substances the IOC demands a full report from the relevant medical authority describing previous drugs tests, subsequent drugs tests and any results of endocrine investigations. If previous tests are unavailable, the results of three, unannounced monthly tests should be included in the report. Failure to cooperate with these proceedings leads to the test being declared as positive.

The side-effects associated with AS use are discussed in Chapter 3.

Testosterone derivatives and androstenedione

These hormones are produced naturally by the body, and are normally present in higher concentrations in males than females.

Beta-2 agonists

Beta-2 agonists may be used in the treatment of asthma and respiratory disorders. These drugs are structurally related to the sympathomimetic amines. They are prohibited by the IOC when administrated orally or by injection. The banned drugs in this category include:

> bambuterol, clenbuterol, fenoterol, fromoterol, reproterol, salbutamol, terbutaline, and related substances.

Salbutamol and terbutaline are permitted if taken by inhalation for the treatment of asthma and/or exercise-induced asthma. Evidence for these conditions must be provided by a team or respiratory physician. This class of drugs stimulates beta-2 receptors in the bronchioli, this stimulation results in dilation of these airways, making it easier for the individual to breathe (Williams, 1997). This is the reason for their use in the therapeutic treatment of asthma.

Beta-2 agonists are classed as stimulants but have been used by some athletes to increase muscle mass. No evidence has been provided with regard to their anabolic potential, and the adverse effects of chronic systemic use of these drugs are, as yet, not fully understood.

Clenbuterol

Clenbuterol is perhaps the best studied drug in this class. It was first banned by the IOC in 1992 following the positive tests of British weightlifters Andrew Saxton and Andrew Davis. These two athletes tested positive for clenbuterol just before the start of the Barcelona Olympics. This drug was banned because its use has been associated with increases in muscle mass and muscle protein synthesis and decreases in body fat. It has been shown that clenbuterol may promote lipolysis (Williams, 1997). Adverse effects reported to be associated with clenbuterol include nervousness, anxiety, tachycardia, palpitations, headaches and insomnia. Most of these effects are considered to be temporary and related to the dose of drug administered (Lenehan, 1997).

1.D. Diuretics

Verroken (1996) states three main reasons for the misuse of diuretics by athletes: to reduce body weight in order to meet weight class limits; to mask the presence of other drugs and their metabolites in the urine; and to overcome fluid retention resulting from use of AS. Diuretics banned by the IOC include:

acetazolamide, bumetanide, chlorthalidone, etacrynic acid, frusemide, hydrochlorthiazide, mannitol, mersalyl, spironolactone, triamterene, and related substances.

Diuretics may offer a potential advantage in sports where there are strict weight class limits (e.g. boxing, weightlifting) or where a slim physique is beneficial. Research by Bradwell *et al.* (1986) suggests that the systemic diuretic, acetazolamide, may improve exercise performance at high altitude.

It should be noted that serious health risks are associated with the misuse of these drugs and there are stringent tests, both in competition and out of competition time, for these drugs. The most serious effects of diuretics misuse are kidney and heart failure, other adverse symptoms include dehydration, faintness, muscle cramps, headaches and nausea.

1.E. Peptide hormones, mimetics and analogues

This doping class was first introduced by the IOC in 1989. The class encompasses a variety of substances with differing applications. The comparatively recent development of some of the drugs in this category, such as synthetic growth hormone, has made this perhaps the most difficult class to test for. The current method of testing for these drugs is by immunoassay (Verroken and Mottram, 1996). Prohibited substances in Class E include the following examples and their analogues and mimetics:

> Chorionic gonadotrophin (human chorionic gonadotrophin, hCG)
> Pituitary and synthetic gonadotrophins (LH)
> Corticotrophin (ACTH, tetracosactide)
> Growth hormone (hGH, somatotrophin)
> Insulin-like growth factor (IGF-1)

and all the respective releasing factors and their analogues.

> Erythropoietin (EPO)
> Insulin – permitted only to treat insulin-dependent diabetes. Written notification of insulin-dependent diabetes by an endocrinologist or team physician is necessary.

If a competitor has an abnormal concentration of an endogenous hormone or its diagnostic marker(s) in their urine, the test is regarded as positive unless it has been conclusively documented to be solely due to a physiological or pathological condition.

Chorionic gonadotrophin (hCG)

This hormone is produced by the placenta and is obtained from the urine of pregnant women. Human chorionic gonadotrophin can be used by males to increase levels of testosterone and epitestosterone; it stimulates the Leydig cells of the testis to produce these two hormones. Following the use of hCG, the urinary excretion of testosterone and epitestosterone is less than the IOC's limit (i.e. a ratio of below 6 : 1 testosterone to epitestosterone); it is believed that this is why abuse of hCG has become popular among athletes (George, 1996a). In addition to the effects of raised testosterone levels, some male athletes may use hCG to prevent testicular atrophy and dysfunction during and after prolonged courses of androgenic drugs such as AS (Kicman *et al.*, 1991).

Side-effects that have been linked with the use of hCG include headaches, tiredness, changes in mood, depression, oedema and a possible link with gynaecomastia (development of female-like breasts in males). Kicman *et al.* (1991) suggest that the occurrence of gynaecomastia in individuals using hCG may be due to raised oestrogen secretion by the testes.

Use of hCG may also have long-term consequences upon the male reproductive system; hCG stimulates testosterone production but suppresses the production of luteinizing hormone releasing factor (LHRF) from the pituitary. This means that when use of hCG ceases there will be low levels of LHRF leading to low levels of LH, giving the overall effect of suppression of testes function.

Pituitary and synthetic gonadotrophins (LH)
Pituitary gonadotrophin (luteinizing hormone, LH) is produced, in males and females, by the gonadotroph cells of the anterior pituitary (George, 1996a). It stimulates testicular sperm production and the synthesis and secretion of testosterone in males. In females, it stimulates ovulation and the production of progesterone. Endogenous regulation of LH is via a negative feedback mechanism whereby secretion of LH is reduced when the levels of testosterone in the plasma are high.

The advantageous effects associated with the use of these drugs are similar to those of anabolic-androgenic steroids and hCG, the raised testosterone levels exerting both anabolic and androgenic effects. Use of LH confers a normal ratio of testosterone to epitestosterone, therefore athletes using LH would not fail the 6 : 1 ratio rule of the IOC. The IOC tests for LH abuse by measuring the ratio of testosterone to LH; tests for normal levels of LH and testosterone are then compared with the samples.

Corticotrophin (ACTH, tetracosactide)
Corticotrophin stimulates the adrenal cortex to secrete corticosteroids. Corticosteroids have been associated with feelings of euphoria and the masking of pain (see section III.D).

Adrenocorticotrophic hormone (ACTH) is a polypeptide made up of 39 amino acids, the N-terminal of the molecule has a vital role in the biological activity of the molecule. This hormone is produced naturally by the corticotroph cells of the anterior pituitary. It stimulates the synthesis and secretion of corticosteroids by the reticularis and fasciculata cells of the adrenal cortex.

Tetracosactrin is the synthetic derivative of ACTH, and therefore also stimulates the production and secretion of corticosteroids such as cortisol and corticosterone. As a result of the decrease in muscle protein synthesis caused by chronic use of ACTH and corticosteroids, wasting of the skeletal muscles may occur. Obviously, this could be particularly detrimental to sporting performance.

A double-blind study by Soetens *et al.* (1995) tested the effects of ACTH upon the performance of 16 professional cyclists. It was discovered that no increase in maximal performance was observed on the day of ACTH intake or the day after ACTH intake. However, self-rated feelings of fatigue were reduced during submaximal performance. Soetens *et al.* also noted that increases in physiological variables such as cortisol, glucose and white corpuscle concentrations were observed in subjects that had received a dose of ACTH. They suggested that the psychological effects of using ACTH could be responsible for the belief that it was a performance-enhancing drug. Despite these findings ACTH is banned by the IOC; this is due to its effect of producing a short-term elevation of plasma cortisol and corticosterone levels. It is suspected that these effects will reduce lethargy and produce positive psychological effects (George, 1996a).

Growth hormone (hGH, somatotrophin)

Tests are currently being developed to detect levels of exogenous growth hormone; these tests are based upon detection of blood markers, including hGH itself and insulin-like growth factor binding proteins (Eichner, 1997).

Human growth hormone has a number of roles in different regulatory processes. It is secreted by the anterior pituitary into the blood supply and is primarily involved in the stimulation of somatic growth in pre-adolescents. However, it also has a number of important roles in the metabolic processes of adults. Exogenous hGH mimics the action of endogenous hGH. Before 1985, hGH was obtained from the pituitary extracts of cadavers. The development of Creutzfeldt–Jakob disease (CJD) in four boys who had been treated with this substance led to the production of genetically engineered growth hormone.

Human growth hormone exerts stimulatory and suppressive effects, its metabolic effects may be acute or delayed. Acute effects last for 3 to 4 hours after physiological doses of growth hormone, delayed effects are exerted after 4 hours.

Evidence for the performance-enhancing qualities of this substance is conflicting (Eichner, 1997). Two studies by Yarasheki *et al.* (1992, 1993) showed that no increases in muscle protein synthesis, muscle size and strength were observed in any of the subjects who had been administered hGH. These studies involved untrained men who had been undergoing a 12-week muscle-building programme and men who were trained weightlifters continuing their training while using hGH. The effects that resulted from the use of hGH included increases in fat-free mass and total body water content, slightly impaired action of insulin, and the development of carpal tunnel syndrome in two men.

However, a study by Papadakis *et al.* (1996) showed that during a 6-month, controlled, double-blind study in which older men (mean age 75 years) were administered hGH, minor increases in lean mass and decreases in fat mass were observed. The group exhibited no improvements in endurance or cognitive function and did not experience any increase in strength.

Adverse effects that have been linked with the misuse of hGH include acromegaly, diabetes mellitus, arthritis and muscle disease (Brisson, 1999). Acromegaly is an irreversible condition characterized by elongation and enlargement of bones of the extremities and certain bones of the head and excessive growth of many organs. In severe cases the effects of this disorder are fairly noticeable, affected individuals have protruding jaws and prominent foreheads and often have coarse, thickened skin. Other effects of acromegaly include visual impairment, muscular weakness, diabetes and decreased libido. There have been reports that a number of athletes already suffer from these symptoms (Cowart, 1988).

Insulin-like growth factor (IGF-1)

Insulin-like growth factor is a relatively recent drug to be used by athletes, it has been traditionally used as a culture medium for cells (Parry, 1996). It is produced endogenously by the liver but has been used as an exogenous drug by athletes to increase anabolism in skeletal muscles. The adverse effects and potential for use as a performance-enhancing drug are still relatively uncertain.

A study by Clemmons (1993) stated that IGF-1 increases anabolism in humans who had been made catabolic as a result of reduced calorie intake. This study also supports the hypothesis that when IGF-1 is used with hGH the anabolic effects are increased.

In a study by Parry (1996) many of the IGF-1 users stated that they were prepared to use this drug while knowing very little, or nothing, about its origins and effects. This presents a cause for concern especially if the use of IGF-1 is to increase within the athletic community.

Erythropoietin

Erythropoietin (EPO) is an endogenous hormone produced by the kidneys. In 1986 a recombinant form of this hormone was developed by scientists at Amgen biotechnology company; this has since been used by athletes primarily for its effect of increasing the oxygen-carrying capability of blood (Pena, 1991). Between the years 1986 and 1991, the deaths of a total of 18 European cyclists were linked with the use of EPO (Pena, 1991). The abuse of this substance seems to be most prevalent in the community of elite cyclists, and this group has suffered the greatest number of losses. Other sports in which abuse of EPO has been reported include endurance sports such as long-distance running and cross-country skiing (Yesalis and Cowart, 1998).

Erythropoietin is attractive as an ergogenic aid because of its ability to increase oxygen transport by the stimulation of red blood cell production by the bone marrow (Ramotar, 1990). Athletes may wish to increase the oxygen-carrying capacity of their blood in an attempt to improve their endurance capacity and recovery times during, and after, competitions (Kicman and Cowan, 1992). It is generally administered by subcutaneous injection and its effects can take 2–3 weeks to manifest themselves (Ramotar, 1990).

It is believed that it is dangerous to have a percentage of red blood cells (haematocrit) of 55% or greater (Yesalis and Cowart, 1998). When the haematocrit becomes this high there is an increased risk of the formation of blood clots, thus considerably increasing the risks of myocardial infarction (heart attack) and cerebrovascular accident (stroke). A high percentage of red blood cells also reduces the speed at which blood travels to vital organs. The risks associated with use of EPO may be increased if strenuous exercise is undertaken, because the dehydrating effects of this type of activity also serve to raise the haematocrit further (Ramotar, 1990). The thickness of the blood may keep on rising for up to 10 days after the last injection of EPO and may remain higher than normal for months (Pena, 1991).

Insulin

A case was reported to the *British Medical Journal* in 1997 of an individual who had used insulin in the belief that it was a highly anabolic substance. This individual sustained severe brain damage after prolonged neuroglycopenia (Elkin *et al.*, 1997). There is no evidence to suggest that this hormone does enhance sporting performance and there are serious risks associated with its abuse.

1.F. Agents with anti-oestrogenic activity

These agents include aromatase inhibitors, clomiphene, cyclofenil and tamoxifen, which are prohibited in males. These drugs are discussed in the following chapter.

1.G. Masking Agents

See section 2.B. below.

PART II. PROHIBITED METHODS

The IOC states that the following methods are prohibited:

2.A. Enhancement of oxygen transfer

Blood doping is defined by the IOC as 'the administration of blood, red blood cells, artificial oxygen carriers and related blood products to an athlete'.

The effects of blood doping are similar to the effects of EPO (described in 1.E.). Blood doping may involve transfusion of a previous sample of the athletes own blood (autologous), or transfusion of blood from a compatible individual (homologous). Athletes may attempt to use this method to improve endurance and to increase aerobic capability by increasing the transport of oxygen to the working muscles (Williams, 1997).

There is conflicting evidence regarding the safety of this method as an ergogenic aid. Williams (1997) states that the method is theoretically safe if carried out under medical supervision and using compatible, screened blood, whereas Verroken (1996) describes serious risks that may be associated with this procedure, including problems with cardiovascular function leading to metabolic shock. A definite risk is involved if the blood used for transfusion is infected with HIV or hepatitis B or C. If incompatible blood from another individual is used for transfusion there is a very serious risk of the occurrence of a potentially fatal haemolytic reaction leading to kidney failure.

2.B. Pharmaceutical, chemical and physical manipulation

Any attempt to alter the integrity or validity of samples used in doping controls by pharmaceutical, chemical or physical manipulation is not permitted by the IOC. Whether the attempt is successful or otherwise is immaterial. The methods that are ruled out include: use of diuretics; alterations of testosterone and epitestosterone[1] measurements (e.g. administration of epitestosterone or bromotan); any methods of catheterization, sample substitution, tampering or inhibition of renal excretion (e.g. use of probnecid).

Urine samples are an effective means to test for the presence of drugs and their metabolites. They are used by the IOC because they provide an easily obtainable, harmless and accurate indication of the drug history of the athlete (Mottram, 1996). The tests employed by the IOC have progressively become more sophisticated and are now able to detect very low levels of banned substances and their metabolites.

The IOC first out-ruled methods of sample manipulation in 1985; the ruling was implemented to prevent competitors from evading positive drugs tests by using samples of 'clean', i.e. drug-free urine. There are reports that competitors may have used the method of pumping drug-free urine into their bladder before giving the sample, a process known as catheterization. The urine used for this method may have been provided by another individual who had not used drugs or may be a sample of the athlete's own urine taken prior to drug use.

Probenecid was added to the list of banned substances in 1987; a test has now been developed for this substance and is used by the IOC. Probnecid delays the excretion of drugs in the urine, which has the effect of prolonging the action of the drug(s) in the body and providing a potential means for the athlete to avoid detection of drugs in their urine sample (Mottram, 1996).

2.C. Gene Doping

Gene or cell doping is defined as the non-therapeutic use of genes, genetic elements and/or cells that have the capacity to enhance performance.

---

[1] An epitestosterone concentration in the urine greater than 200 nanograms per millilitre will be investigated by studies (see section 1.C.).

PART III. CLASSES OF DRUGS SUBJECT TO CERTAIN RESTRICTIONS

3.A. Alcohol

Tests are conducted by the IOC for ethanol. Alcohol may be used by athletes to combat anxiety (Reilly, 1996). It is classed as a depressant and its effects on the central nervous system tend to be proportional to the blood concentration (Wadler and Hainline, 1989). Previous studies have shown that ethanol can produce a number of neuronal changes including reduction of the sodium current underlying the action potential, changes in resting permeability and active transport, and changes in the postsynaptic excitory current (Wallgren and Barry, 1970; Zornetzer *et al.*, 1982).

Reilly (1996) states that a number of problems are encountered when attempting to carry out a controlled study of the effects of alcohol on exercise. First, it is difficult to perform 'blind', i.e. placebo-controlled, experiments because the subjects will be likely to recognize the taste of alcohol. To overcome this problem researchers have used placebos containing minimal quantities of alcohol, usually in the form of vodka mixed with orange juice. Minimal levels of alcohol should not produce measurable concentrations of alcohol in the blood but still give the subject the impression that they have consumed some alcohol.

Other problems outlined by Reilly (1996) include problems regarding the different responses of subjects to alcohol, and differences in the levels of blood alcohol induced. Most experiments use levels of alcohol that are in accordance with the body weights of their subjects. This is because the effects that alcohol exerts on the individual vary depending on body size.

The exact effects of alcohol on sporting performance are still to be determined but it is known that performance parameters including maximum oxygen uptake, oxygen consumption, and aerobic capacity are unaffected by moderate doses of alcohol (Hebbellinck, 1959, 1963; Williams, 1969; Wadler and Hainline, 1989).

It is generally believed that moderate levels of anxiety may improve motivation and thereby enhance performance. However, when an individual is over-anxious the effects on performance are most often adverse. Alcohol is easy to obtain and more socially acceptable than most of the other 'banned' drugs, it is therefore unsurprising that some athletes use it to overcome their anxiety. It is potentially addictive and is associated with a number of adverse effects, which may be direct or indirect. Direct effects on sporting performance include impaired hand–eye coordination, slower simple reaction time, impaired judgment and reduced coordination. Indirect effects may be related to social factors or the residual effects exerted by heavy drinking upon subsequent training sessions or competitions (Reilly, 1996).

Shooting and aiming sports have been most frequently associated with the use of alcohol to aid performance (Reilly, 1996). It was discovered by

Koller and Biary (1984) that alcohol, in moderate doses, was better than propanolol in controlling postural essential tremor. Reilly (1996) also states that low doses of alcohol may improve the steadiness of the arm in activities such as archery, darts and pistol shooting. Steadiness of aim and judgement are not improved by moderate doses of alcohol.

Chronic alcohol abuse is associated with many serious health problems. It has adverse effects on the central and peripheral nervous systems, cardio-vascular function, liver function and general mental health.

3.B. Cannabinoids

Tests are conducted for cannabinoids such as marijuana. Urine samples containing greater than 15 nanograms per millilitre of 11-nor-delta-9-tetrahydrocannabinol-9-carboxylic acid (carboxy-THC) are deemed positive.

Delta-9-tetrahydrocannabinol (delta-9-THC) is the main active constituent of the cannabis plant. This substance has effects on the central nervous system and has influences on several different neurochemical pathways. The effects from smoking marijuana include decreased motivation for physical effort, decreased motor coordination, decrease in the ability of short-term recall, and changes in perception (Reilly, 1996). Wadler and Hainline (1989) state that the acute effects of marijuana are reported to last for 4 hours.

The specific effects that are potentially detrimental to performance in most sports include impaired hand–eye coordination and fast reaction time (Borg, 1973; Reilly, 1996). Other effects have also been linked with de-creased sporting performance; Renaud and Cormier (1986) discovered that after smoking marijuana the maximal work capacity is decreased and the maximal heart rate is achieved at a lower intensity during a graded exercise.

Much controversy surrounds the psychological effects of marijuana, and whether it is physically addictive is still unclear. Some studies have shown that it induces the 'amotivational syndrome' (Smith, 1968; Hollister, 1986), which is characterized by general apathy towards future plans and impaired judgement. Further research is necessary to establish the validity of this 'syndrome' and the possible implications it may have upon athletic performance.

3.C. Local anaesthetics

The IOC permits the use of certain injectable local anaesthetics, but specific conditions are outlined for their use. The use of cocaine as a local anaesthetic and the administration of local anaesthetics by systemic injection are not permitted by the IOC.

Bupivacaine, lidocaine, mepivacaine and procaine may be used but only by local or intra-articular injections. Vasoconstrictor agents, such as adrena-line, are allowed to be used in conjunction with the local anaesthetics previ-ously mentioned. It is specified that these substances may only be used when medically justified.

The IOC implemented these measures to control the misuse of these drugs by athletes. These drugs are used to treat injuries and block pain. If an athlete uses local anaesthetics to mask the pain of an injury, and then continues to train, there is an increased risk of further injury because the normal pain threshold has been masked (Verroken, 1996). The injection of any drug is associated with certain risks; clean needles and good hygiene procedures should always be used to reduce the risk of infection. The repeated intra-articular injection of local anaesthetics has also been associated with local arthropathy (joint problems) (Haynes and Murad, 1985).

3.D. Glucocorticosteroids

The anal, aural, dermatological, inhalation, nasal and ophthalmological administration of these substances is permitted by the IOC. Oral, systemic injections and rectal administration of these drugs is not permitted. Intra-articular and local injections are allowed but, again, notification of any of the types of administration may be required.

Corticosteroids are produced naturally in the body by the adrenal cortex. They are not responsible for the initiation of cellular and enzymatic activity but they enable certain reactions in the body to occur at optimal rates.

Synthetic corticosteriods are primarily anti-inflammatory drugs. They may be misused by athletes in large doses in attempt to mask injury and to enhance athletic ability. They may be used in smaller doses by athletes as bronchodilators. Medically, they are used to treat asthma and as anti-inflammatory pain relievers. They tend to be used most frequently as topical preparations because they are associated with adverse symptoms, but also euphoria, when used systemically. They are also potentially toxic if used for long periods of time without medical supervision.

3.E. Beta blockers

Specific examples of beta blockers banned by the IOC include:

> acebutolol, alprenolol, atenolol, labetolol, metoprolol, nadolol, oxprenolol, propanolol, sotalol and related substances.

Beta blockers (also known as beta-adrenergic blockers) are generally used by the medical profession for the treatment of cardiovascular disorders and hypertension. They tend to be used in sports to reduce anxiety and to steady the arms and hands. They exert the effect of slowing down the heart rate by acting to inhibit the actions of epinephrine and norepinephrine (Williams, 1997). Beta blockers act upon beta receptors at different sites in the body; the heart rate is slowed down when they act upon the beta receptors of the heart.

These drugs may have the potential to cause symptoms that are potentially detrimental to sporting performance. Specific examples include sleep disturbances and cold hands (Goldman, 1984). Other potentially adverse effects that may be experienced with misuse of beta blockers include low blood pressure, sexual dysfunction and central nervous system depressive symptoms.

4.10 *World Anti-Doping Agency (WADA)*

Through an initiative led by the International Olympic Committee, following the debacle of the 1998 Tour de France, WADA was created in November 1999 to support and promote fundamental values in sport. It is an attempt to unify sport and harmonize the way in which individual sport organisations as well as nations approach the fight against doping. Apart from regular, at least annual, reviews of the prohibited drug list, it will also attempt to harmonize the way in which samples are taken and analysed. To facilitate its work the WADA has introduced a World Anti-Doping Code. The Code will harmonize rules and regulations regarding doping across all countries and all sports in an attempt to create a level playing field for athletes. The aim is to have the Code in place, and ratified by a large number of countries, for the Olympic Games in Athens in 2004.

One of the initiatives is the introduction of the Athlete Passport. An integral part of its anit-doping programme and a requirement in the World Anti-Doping Code is for athletes to provide accurate, up to date information about their whereabouts.

4.11 *Summary*

Some athletes want to use drugs. Those who are subjected to IOC dope-testing controls cannot use drugs without running the risk of being banned for life from their sport. But the original idea of urine controls, of weeding out the use of substances such as anabolic steroids, was based on concerns for the health of the athletes after several highly publicized deaths, such as that of cyclist Tommy Simpson. Ben Johnson's coach, Charlie Francis, is in no doubt about the success of the dope testers. 'If the IOC and IAAF drug policies were designed to protect the athletes' health, they have failed . . . Moral outrage has short-circuited the scientific method . . . Rather than inducing people to perform without drugs, the banned list has pushed them up the endocrine ladder to new substances with harsher side effects or unknown risks, there are concerns that this shall lead to a race to find new undetectable ergogenic and masking substance. In this context, the demonization of steroids has done no-one a favour . . . Today's athlete is forced to seek not the safest effective drugs but the ones that are least detectable' (Francis, 1990).

CHAPTER 5

Regimes, counterfeits and profiles

Anabolic steroids are generally self-administered, often in large super-therapeutic dosages (Korkia and Stimson, 1993; Lenehan *et al.*, 1996; Evans, 1997). The majority of users 'stack' AS, that is the taking of two or more different drugs at the same time; the number of drugs taken can be as low as two or as high as 16 (Korkia and Stimson, 1993; Lenehan *et al.*, 1996). Lists and descriptions of AS, their effectiveness and common side-effects as reported by users themselves can be found in many of the 'underground handbooks' that have become commonplace in the AS-using culture over the past 10 years (Philips, 1991). The drugs are generally taken in cycles which, for men, often vary from 8 to 12 weeks on-AS followed by 8 to 12 weeks off-AS. 'Female' cycles tend to be shorter, often half of those reported by men (Korkia and Stimson, 1993). 'Cycling' AS attempts to maximize gains while minimizing their harmful effects. Anabolic steroids work through a receptor complex and once these get saturated the drug will not have any further beneficial effect but instead will contribute to the development of side-effects. Within a cycle a large number of different AS may be used but not necessarily all at the same time. Some drugs are generally preferred at different stages of the 'cycle' depending on what the user aims to achieve, for instance, 'cutting', 'size', 'strength', 'bulking', 'maintenance' or 'muscle hardness'.

Polypharmacy is common among AS users. The fact that AS are not used by themselves but with a number of other drugs and supplements makes the evaluation of their efficacy and that of adverse effects very complicated. In order to potentiate the effects of AS, many users are prepared to use concomitant drugs. It is hoped by the user that the use of another drug may increase the ability to train by increasing the effort involved, increasing the time they are able to workout, and decreasing the time required to recover between workouts. Other drugs may be used to counteract the side-effects of steroids so that the body will be able to tolerate higher or longer doses of AS.

Various chemical substances have been used as additional drugs, including caffeine, ephedrine, amphetamines, cocaine, clenbuterol, insulin, Nubain and growth hormone. Diet manipulation may also be attempted by taking large quantities of nutritional supplements (Clarkson, 1996).

Many AS users believe that some drugs work synergistically, and the 'underground' steroid handbooks provide numerous examples of these regimes. Many of these regimes are purely the personal opinion of the authors of these books, often the result of trial and error rather than scientific study. However, they often are considered to be facts by AS users purely because they appear in print. Although AS are generally taken in cycles, some people use them continuously, while some take 'maintenance' dosages while 'off' AS to prevent an excessive decline in muscle mass.

It is common for AS to be taken in vast excess of recommended therapeutic dosages. Kochakian and Endahl suggested in 1959 that side-effects are dose related. Dosages can be 34 times the recommended therapeutic dose (Korkia and Stimson, 1993). Evans (1997) reported that 88% of the 100 AS users in his sample took two or more drugs during a cycle and 50% took a weekly dose of 500 mg or less, while 35% took between 500 and 1000 mg and the remaining 12% took in excess of 1000 mg per week: the minimum and maximum doses were 250 and 3200 mg, respectively. Many AS users are unaware of the amount of AS that they are actually using or sometimes even what drug they are using. This problem can be compounded by the fact that AS often come in a variety of doses; for example, nandrolone decanoate comes in 25, 50, 100 and 200 milligrams per millilitre. Another factor that can have a considerable bearing on the dose used are the fakes and counterfeits that are commonly available to AS users; this is discussed in more detail later. Millar (1994, 1996) has treated AS users for the past 15 years in Australia and he believes that AS can be administered in far lower doses than currently used by strength athletes with good gains and no particular side-effects. He has been prescribing no more than 500 mg per week for up to 9 weeks.

5.1 *Cost*

The cost of an AS 'cycle' was reported to be on average about £70 (£13–£500) by Korkia and Stimson (1993) and £140 (£15–£2000) by Lenehan *et al.* (1996). Body-builders and weightlifters from 14 different gyms in London and the Bournemouth area reported spending between £500 and £2500 annually on performance-enhancing drugs, amounting to 45% of the total cost of training (Parry, 1996). Evans' (1997) interviewees spent between £40 and £370 during a typical 4-week period on AS.

5.2 *Counterfeits and fakes*

The existence of counterfeit AS is by no means a new phenomenon. Because of the limited availability of genuine pharmaceutical products and the laws of supply and demand, many AS users have grown to accept the fact that the majority of products available to them will be either fake or counterfeit. However, it is important to note that although the terms fake and counterfeit may imply inferior quality, there is evidence to suggest that many of these products do in fact contain AS (although not always of the dosage or type specified). In some instances these products have acquired such a positive reputation that they have become sought after in their own right, even to the extent of being counterfeited themselves.

Traditionally, fake AS were relatively easy to identify if you knew what to look for. Poor packaging, badly printed or photocopied information inserts and bar codes that often appeared to have been drawn with a felt-tip pen (and in some cases had been) were and still are the most obvious indications of fake products. Other pointers include visible contamination of ampoules, variability in appearance and content of ampoules and vials, and incorrect tablet consistency. There are, however, exceptions to these guidelines as is evident in the poor quality packaging of genuine pharmaceutical products manufactured in developing countries. While it is still possible to find these rather amateurish fakes being sold to the unwary, a more sophisticated type of product has appeared on the market that is much more difficult to identify.

One of the most disturbing aspects of fake and counterfeit AS is the variation in content of these products. This is especially significant when one considers that some AS that have been tested were found to contain nearly twice the strength of the stated content (McVeigh and Lenehan, 1994). These results clearly demonstrate the problems facing AS users who purchase products on the illicit market. Many users will be aware of the probability of a product being fake or counterfeit. There is often the presumption that the fake steroid will be weaker than the stated content. The user will often compensate for this by increasing the amount taken, a highly dangerous practice.

In addition to the strength variations of illicitly produced AS, there are many examples of the stated AS being substituted with a different active ingredient. There have been cases of high androgenic steroids being packaged as steroids with much lower androgenic properties. Many of the side-effects associated with AS are a direct result of their androgenic properties. The potential for harm can be greatly increased if large doses of high androgenic steroids are used. The risk to female AS users is particularly worrying as the virilizing effect of androgens in women may result in irreversible side-effects.

Ritsch and Musshoff (2000) evaluated 40 AS obtained from the German black market and found that 37.5% of the drugs contained different or none of the pharmacological compounds labelled. In Merseyside, McVeigh and Lenehan (1994) had four AS tested. Although all contained some AS, they varied from 43% to 73% of their stated content. In response to the concerns about the prevalence and dangers of counterfeit AS, the Welsh Office funded a study that enabled the purchase and analysis of black market products (Perry, 1995). Again, a vast discrepancy between actual and labelled incredients was found: four different brands of nandrolone, three brands of methandienone, four brands of stanozolol and four samples of testosterone all contained somewhere between 0 and 169% of the stated content. The investigator highlighted several key issues:

1 Danger of overdosing, especially relevant for women who strive to avoid the androgenic effects of the drug.
2 Sterility of injectable drugs (there were reports of sunflower cooking oil having been used instead of arachis oil).
3 Two samples of the same drug from the same 'manufacturer' contained differing amounts of AS.

An extreme case of the dangers of the black market supply is described by Perry and Hughes (1992). A 30-year-old AS user had acquired haldol decanoate from the black market in the belief that it was the commonly used AS nandrolone decanoate. He developed acute depression and suicidal ideas, and continued to have psychiatric problems for at least 9 months.

There are problems regarding the provision of information about fakes and counterfeits. It must be emphasized that information on the contents of drugs that have been tested relate only to the specific substance tested, it must not be presumed that a product of identical appearance will necessarily have the same contents. Fake steroids will often use the same batch number all the time. This means that different batches with potentially different amounts of active ingredients will always look the same.

5.3 *Drugs other than anabolic steroids*

In order to potentiate the effects of AS many users are prepared to use concomitant drugs. It is hoped by the user that the use of another drug may increase the ability to train by increasing the effort involved, increasing the time they are able to workout, and decreasing the time required to recover between workouts. Other drugs may be used to counteract the side-effects of steroids so that the body will be able to tolerate higher or longer doses of AS.

Various chemical substances have been used as additional drugs, including caffeine, ephedrine, amphetamines, cocaine, clenbuterol, insulin, Nubain and growth hormone, as well as large quantities of nutritional supplements (Clarkson, 1996).

Caffeine is widely used as a mild stimulant and has been found to increase vigilance, reaction times and feelings of well-being and enhances long-term endurance exercise (Rogers *et al.*, 1995). It is suggested that caffeine has a direct effect on calcium exchange by the sarcoplasmic reticulum or inhibits phosphodiesterase or is an adenosine receptor antagonist, which causes increased muscle strength by enhanced neuromuscular transmission and muscle fibre contractility (Doherty, 1996). Optimal doses appear to be between 100 and 200 mg. Side-effects that could be encountered are irritability, insomnia, peptic ulcers and cardiac arrhythmias.

Carnitine has become popular as a nutritional supplement and is widely used by those who would not consider using AS. Carnitine's main role is to transport long-chain fatty acids from the cytosol to the mitochondria by beta-oxidation. This mechanism becomes the main source of energy for the muscles in endurance exercising and an increase in carnitine may spare glycogen, so delaying fatigue. There are no reported adverse effects to date but the theoretical potential of enhancing the metabolism is doubtful (Heinonen, 1996).

Creatine has been used for short-term exercise as it is suggested that the creatine will be stored as creatine phosphate in the muscle and therefore ready to release energy by mitochondrial ATP synthesis. The phosphate may also act as a buffer for lactic acid, so increasing the rate of recovery after exercise. Again the effects of this supplement are largely discounted in the medical literature (Thompson *et al.*, 1996) but there are no significant adverse effects reported.

Phenylpropanolamine and ephedrine are easily available over the counter in chemists as ingredients in cold and influenza remedies. Although commonly used there are no scientific data supporting these compounds as ergogenic aids. Adverse effects include hypertension, headaches, dizziness and tachycardia (Wadler and Hainline, 1989).

A more potent sympathomimetic drug is amphetamine. It has powerful stimulating effects on the central nervous system such as increased excitation and euphoria at the expense of misjudgments in coordination. Some studies suggest there is a marginal benefit to AS users in performance that is outweighed by the possible side-effects, which include heat-stroke after intense exercise. The psychoactive nature of this drug can lead to psychological dependence and depression during drug withdrawal.

Cocaine is thought to have greater addictive properties. It is used to increase vigour and endurance, decrease tiredness, and promote euphoria and greater motor activity. Cocaine use is associated with cerebrovascular accidents caused by either spasm or rupture of blood vessels in the brain. Cocaine combined with alcohol ingestion increases the risks of cardiotoxicity by the production of a metabolite cocaethylene (Morrison, 1996).

Clenbuterol is a beta-2 agonist used medically as an inhaled aerosol to counteract bronchial constriction in the treatment of asthma. Animal studies have shown that clenbuterol increases skeletal muscle mass and reduces body fat. Its misuse has become widespread recently and it is readily available. In the livestock industry beta-2 agonists have been used to some success in increasing lean muscle mass and reducing adipose disposition and this has led to its popularity in the illicit AS-using market. The pharmacodynamic effects of clenbuterol have yet to be established, with studies producing conflicting data. However, it is believed that clenbuterol increases the rate of muscle protein deposition and promotes lipolysis in skeletal and cardiac muscle only. It exerts a suppressive effect on protein degradation and increases the intramuscular concentration of proteolytic proteinase inhibitors.

The growth-enhancing effect of clenbuterol reduces with chronic use and appears to be of a time-limited value as a result of the downregulation of receptor numbers and responsiveness. Severe side-effects have been reported in AS users, including adrenergic tremor and tachycardia. Two deaths have resulted due to ignorance of safe doses and so overdose has occurred (Prather *et al.*, 1995).

Some AS users are now beginning to use insulin, which has been readily available without prescriptions at chemists. Although it has been well established in scientific research that insulin is a strong anabolic agent (Russell-Jones and Umpleby, 1996), it has only recently become an increasing drug-use trend in AS users. Its popularity may be as a result of competitive athletes trying to circumvent detection by the dope-testing agencies looking for AS misuse. When this happens these drug trends will eventually trickle down to the non-athlete, recreational AS user. Normal physiological function would easily compensate for small doses of insulin administered to a healthy individual but use by a non-trained person could lead to excessive amounts given, leading to hypoglycaemic coma and severe brain damage (Elkin *et al.*, 1997) or even death. Insulin has a positive effect on albumin synthesis and has an important anabolic role during nutrient absorption by promoting uptake of relevant amounts of dietary amino acids into the proteins. Insulin cannot exert any anabolic action in muscle if there is insufficient amino acid availability. Insulin promotes protein anabolism by reducing the rates of amino acid oxidation and endogenous proteolysis but does not increase protein synthesis at a whole-body level.

Growth hormone (GH) is produced by the anterior pituitary and is used medically as a replacement in children who are deficient in this hormone and in the treatment of children with delayed growth and short children due to intrauterine growth retardation. Growth hormone is one of the important influences on the speed and activation of somatic growth and development in children; it can cause an increase in the length of muscle fibres, and in adults the diameter. The function of GH is to promote the production of insulin-like growth factor. Both promote anabolism causing muscle, bone and cartilage growth. Increased protein deposition occurs due to increased amino acid uptake and protein synthesis in cells with an associated reduction in protein catabolism. Growth hormone-induced growth is different to work-induced growth as GH causes an increase in the rate and translation of existing RNA, whereas work-related growth requires the synthesis of new RNA. It has been demonstrated that exogenous GH will increase fat-free weight and decrease the percentage of body fat following a 6-week course of resistance exercises (Crist *et al.*, 1988).

More AS users are adding GH to their menu of drugs despite levels of GH being elevated by AS (Haupt, 1993). Exogenous GH could mimic the signs of acromegaly with associated myopathy and peripheral neuropathy and could produce symptoms such as prognathism, protrusion of the jaw bone caused by periosteal overgrowth and cortical thickening. Hands are widened and fingers become broadened. Erosion of the surfaces of joints occurs with polymyalgia. Soft-tissue thickening leads to coarsening of the facial features. The internal organs also enlarge, especially the heart. Biochemical effects include glucose intolerance leading to hyperglycaemia and hyperlipidaemia. Arthritis, impotence and thickening of the skin occur. Overgrowth of organs and tissues associated with excessive use of GH is probably permanent. The appearance of acromegaly in an AS user also self-administering GH has not yet been reported.

Insulin-like growth factor I (IGF-I) has more recently appeared on the AS drug-user scene. It is essentially used in laboratories for research and has very limited use within a clinical setting but seems to be available on the illicit market (Parry, 1996). IGF-I is an endocrine hormone that attenuates the effects of GH and when used in combination is substantially more anabolic than either used alone. It increases energy expenditure and lipid oxidation and decreases proteolysis and protein oxidation. IGF-I is especially anabolic for skeletal muscle but whereas GH has a tendency to cause hyperglycaemia, with IGF-I hypoglycaemia can be problematic as insulin sensitivity is increased. Oedema and jaw pain are other reported side-effects.

Human chorionic gonadotrophin (hCG) is produced in the human placenta during pregnancy but when injected into males it mimics the effects of luteinizing hormone, so stimulating natural testosterone production from the testes. Non-competitive AS users use this compound during drug-free intervals between cycles in an attempt to restimulate the normal sex hormone production and function of the testes, which was suppressed by the megadoses of endogenous AS. In sportsmen hCG has become popular in an attempt to circumvent AS detection in doping investigations (Kicman *et al.*, 1991). hCG has been implicated as having an increased risk of producing gynaecomastia.

Erythropoietin (EPO) is mainly used by endurance athletes as a doping mechanism to increase aerobic endurance prior to competition and so leads to no perceived benefits for the body-sculpting AS user. EPO is a glycoprotein produced by the kidney and a smaller proportion by the liver that regulates red blood cell production and is medically used in the treatment of certain anaemias. The resultant increase in red blood cells will lead to a higher oxygen-carrying capacity for the athlete. Hypertension and hyperviscosity of the blood leading to a thromboembolic event secondary to sludging of the blood are reported side-effects that could be life threatening (Thein *et al.*, 1995).

Because of the purchasing power of AS users suppliers have been able to obtain any sort of medication that is believed to be the best in its category. Nubain had been widely used as an effective painkiller for muscular injuries in AS users who want to continue training despite their injuries. Users have been unaware of the drug's opioid characteristics and dependence on this drug has been reported (McBride *et al.*, 1996).

5.4 *Drug profiles*

This information has been gleaned from a number of sources over many years. Where the term 'street information' has been used it refers to information gathered from the many 'underground' handbooks that are available or from information supplied by users of AS and related drugs. I have deliberately left out common dosages used by AS users in case they were misinterpreted as recommended amounts as they are often many times a therapeutic dose. Where possible I have included therapeutic dosages that might be prescribed by physicians for illnesses. However, many of these substances do not have recognized therapeutic uses and therefore no dose can be given.

5.4.1 NANDROLONE DECANOATE (INJECTABLE)

Alternative names:

Nortestosterone decanoate
Nortestosterone decylate

Proprietary names:

Anaboline (50 mg/mL)
Anabolin LA-100
Deca-Durabol (25, 50, 100 mg/mL)
Deca-Durabolin (25, 50, 100, 200 mg/mL)
Dece-Ject (25, 50 mg/mL)
Elpihormo (50 mg/mL)
Extraboline (50 mg/mL)
Hybolin decanoate (50, 100 mg/mL)

Jebolan (50 mg/mL)
Nandrolone decanoate
  (50, 100, 200 mg/mL)
Nurezan (50 mg/mL)
Retabolil (25, 50 mg/mL)
Retabolin (50 mg/mL)
Turinabol Depot (50 mg/mL)
Ziremilon (50 mg/mL)

Veterinary products:

Anabolicum
Norandren

Therapeutic dose:

50 mg every 3 weeks (osteoporosis in post-menopausal women)
50–100 mg weekly (aplastic anaemia)

Nandrolone decanoate in the form of the Organon product, Deca-Durabolin, has been around for over 30 years. It has anabolic, androgenic, progestogenic and erythropoietic activity. The steroid maintains the anabolic activity of testosterone but the androgenic action is markedly diminished. The anabolic/androgenic quotient after 2 weeks of treatment has been shown to be 12 times that obtained with testosterone decanoate. Nandrolone decanoate has been shown to influence calcium metabolism positively and to increase bone mass in osteoporosis. Androgenic effects are relatively uncommon at the recommended therapeutic dosages.

As nandrolone is not C17-alpha-alkylated it does not have as strong an association with the occurrence of liver dysfunction and cholestasis. However, it may cause fluid retention and oedema due to sodium retention by the kidney. Nandrolone decanoate is slowly released from the injection site into the blood with a half-life of 6–8 days.

Nandrolone decanoate has been used to treat a variety of disorders, including:

osteoporosis in post-menopausal women
disseminated breast cancer in women
protein deficiency states occurring after major surgery or trauma
anaemia
chronic renal failure

Street information
Nandrolone decanoate (Deca) is widely considered to be the most commonly used injectable AS for performance enhancement. It also has the reputation for being one of the most frequently detected banned substances (metabolites can be detected for periods in excess of one year). Because of its popularity Deca has been widely counterfeited, and because of its relatively low androgenic properties it is also commonly thought to aromatize only at high doses. Deca is commonly used for 'bulking-up' and has a reputation for promoting size and strength. There have also been reports of Deca being effective in alleviating joint and tendon pains. Although some body-builders have found Deca effective during the pre-competition phase, others have found water retention to be a problem. Reports of side-effects include hypertension, acne,

and sexual and reproductive problems. The occurrence of side-effects appears to be more common in females and is influenced strongly by the dosage used. The most common incidences of adverse effects include facial hair growth, deepening of the voice and clitoral enlargement.

5.4.2 METHANDROSTENOLONE (ORAL)

Alternative names:

Methandienone
Metandienone

Proprietary names:

Anabol (5 mg)   Metanabol (1 mg/5 mg)
Andoredan (5 mg)   Methandrostenolonum (5 mg)
Bionabol (2 mg/5 mg)   Naposim (5 mg)
Encephan (5 mg)   Nerobol (5 mg)
Metabol (5 mg)   Pronabol (5 mg)
Metaboline (also contains multivitamins   Stenolon (1 mg/5 mg)
and nutrients) (5 mg)   Trinergic (5 mg capsules)

Veterinary/Injectable: 25 mg/mL

Anabolikum
Metandiabol

Therapeutic dose:

4 mg orally daily (pain relief in osteoporosis), 6 weeks on, 4 weeks off

Methandrostenolone, usually referred to as Dianabol, was first produced and marketed by Ciba-Geigy in 1960. It was promoted as being highly anabolic, androgenic, with little progestational activity. Dianabol was also reported to enhance feelings of well-being. Dianabol was indicated for the treatment of disorders requiring increased protein synthesis and osteoporosis. Dianabol has a relatively short half-life, between 3.2 and 4.5 hours, with maximum blood concentration occurring between 1 and 3 hours. Methandrostenolone and methandienone are almost identical, the only difference being in the spatial configuration of their chemical structure. They are 17-alpha-alkylated compounds and therefore exert a significant strain on the liver, with even relatively low dosages causing temporary abnormalities in liver function tests. There have been reports of the development of jaundice being attributed to methandrostenolone/methandienone and there have also been cases of liver carcinoma and adenoma associated with its use.

Street information

Many users of this steroid have reported dramatic gains in both strength and size. However, it aromatizes even at low dosages, with the development of gynaecomastia a common problem. Another common complaint is the problem of water retention, resulting in hypertension. As methandrostenolone has a high level of conversion to dihydrotestosterone the development of acne vulgaris is common, as is the acceleration of male pattern baldness in those with an hereditary predisposition. Female use of methandrostenolone can result in virilization due to its androgenic properties. Masculinizing effects can occur even at low dosages in some women who are particularly sensitive to androgens.

5.4.3 OXANDROLONE (ORAL)

Proprietary names:

Anavar (2.5 mg)	Oxandrin (2.5 mg)
Lipidex (2.5 mg)	Vasorome (2.5 mg)
Lonavar (2 mg)	

Oxandrolone is rapidly absorbed from the gastrointestinal tract, resulting in a maximum plasma concentration between 30 and 90 minutes and a plasma half-life of about 9 hours. Oxandrolone has been given orally in the treatment of constitutional delayed growth and puberty in boys. Courses of treatment are short (about 3 to 4 months) because of the risk of epiphyseal closure. Oxandrolone has been prescribed to post-menopausal women in the treatment of osteoporosis. Oxandrolone is also under investigation in the treatment of Turner's syndrome in girls. As oxandrolone is C17-alpha-alkylated there is the potential for liver damage.

Street information

Oxandrolone has relatively low androgenic properties, with little aromatization in males. It has a reputation for increasing strength but not size. It is popular with women because of its low incidence of side-effects due to virilization, but some cases of facial hair growth and deepening of the voice have been reported following prolonged dosages. Gastrointestinal irritation, including pain and diarrhoea, are commonly reported side-effects in both male and female users.

5.4.4 OXYMETHOLONE (ORAL)

Proprietary names:

Adroyd (50 mg)	Oxitosona (50 mg)
Anadrol 50 (50 mg)	Plenastril (50 mg)
Anapolon (5 mg)	Roborol (50 mg)
Anapalon 50 (50 mg)	Synasteron (50 mg)
Hemogenin (50 mg)	

Therapeutic dose:

1–5 mg per kg of body weight daily

Oxymetholone has anabolic and androgenic properties. It is used orally in the treatment of anaemias such as aplastic anaemias. Oxymetholone is 17-alpha-alkylated, with liver disturbances and jaundice common even at therapeutic doses. There have also been links between oxymetholone treatment and the development of leukaemia.

Street information
Oxymetholone, a derivative of dihydrotestosterone (DHT), is commonly recognized as the strongest oral AS available. It is both highly anabolic and androgenic and, being 17-alpha-alkylated, very toxic to the liver. There have been many reports of acne and hair loss (due to high levels of DHT) in addition to its strong association with liver damage and gynaecomastia. There have also been reports of headaches and stomach pains. There is substantial evidence of loss of size and weight, which has been attributed to the drug being too hard on the body. Very few women are able to tolerate oxymetholone because of its virilizing effects.

5.4.5 METHENOLONE ACETATE (ORAL)

Alternative names:

Metenolone acetate

Proprietary names:

Primobolan (5 mg)
Primobolan S (25 mg)

Primobolan has been on the market for over 30 years. The injection form of the acetate has been discontinued, but the tablet form is still available.

Methenolone acetate is not licensed for use in the UK, but has been used on occasion overseas, mainly for its anabolic action. It has moderate anabolic properties and a low androgenic component. Primobolan tablets are not C17-alpha-alkylated and do not have the liver toxicity associated with many of the other oral AS.

Street information
Primobolan has a reputation for having low androgenic properties causing little aromatization, water retention or liver damage. It is generally considered to be one of the safest AS. Muscle gains are reported to be slow to develop but of good quality. Primobolan is popular with competitive body-builders as a pre-contest drug, as it is believed that it causes little water retention, and with women because of its relatively low androgenic properties.

5.4.6 METHENOLONE ENANTHATE (INJECTABLE)

Alternative names:

Metenolone enantate
Metenolone enanthate
Methenolone oenanthate

Proprietary names:

Primobolan Depot (50 mg/mL, 100 mg/mL)

Methenolone enanthate is the long-acting injectable version of Primobolan tablets (methenolone acetate).

Street information
Primobolan Depot has a reputation for having low androgenic properties causing little aromatization, water retention or liver damage. It is generally considered to be a much milder AS than nandrolone decanoate.

5.4.7 STANOZOLOL (ORAL)

Alternative names:

Androstanazole
Methylstanazole

Proprietary names:

Stromba (5 mg)
Winstrol (2 mg)

Therapeutic dose:

2.5–10 mg daily

Stanozolol has anabolic and androgenic properties and has been used in the treatment of vascular manifestations of Behçet's syndrome and in the management of hereditary angio-oedema. Stanozolol, when given for prolonged periods, has been associated with elevated liver function results as it is a 17-alpha-alkylated compound.

Street information
Stanozolol tablets have a reputation for causing gastrointestinal discomfort after prolonged use. Both the tablets and the injection form are not considered to aromatize. Tablets are often taken in divided doses to reduce the gastric irritation. This practice is popular with female users, as it reduces the risks of virilization that is associated with large amounts of androgens in the female system.

5.4.8 Stanozolol (Injectable)

Alternative names:

Androstanazole
Methylstanazole

Proprietary names:

Stromba (50 mg/mL)
Stromaject (50 mg/mL)
Winstrol Depot (50 mg/mL)

Veterinary product:

Winstrol V (50 mg/mL)

Stanozolol is considered by many steroid users to have relatively low androgenic properties. As it is a water-based, injectable steroid, it has a relatively short half-life.

Street information
The injectable versions of Stanozolol (both human and veterinary) are far more popular than the tablet forms. Although gains are considered to be achieved slowly with this product, its low incidence of water retention makes it popular as a pre-contest drug. Stromba has a reputation for being

fast-acting and quickly excreted from the body, as it is water based rather than oil based. Therefore, it is common to find it being injected several times a week.

5.4.9 SUSTANON 250 (INJECTABLE)

Alternative names:

Sostenon 250
Sustenon 250

Veterinary products:

Deposterone

Therapeutic dose:

1 mL every 3 weeks

Sustanon contains four different testosterones:

Testosterone propionate	30 mg
Testosterone phenylpropionate	60 mg
Testosterone isocaproate	60 mg
Testosterone decanoate	100 mg

Sustanon 250 has considerable anabolic and androgenic properties. It was designed to maximize the synergistic effect of using four testosterones. The variation in half-life times of the testosterones means that the product is fast-acting and remains effective for several weeks. Total plasma testosterone levels peak approximately 24–48 hours after administration. Plasma testosterone levels return to the lower limit of the normal range in males in approximately 21 days. Sustanon is predominantly used as testosterone replacement therapy in the treatment of male hypogonadal disorders such as eunuchoidism (following castration), hypopituitarism, endocrine impotence, decreased libido and disorders of spermatogenesis. Testosterone therapy may also be indicated for the prevention and treatment of osteoporosis in hypogonadal males.

Street information
Sustanon 250 has a reputation for being very effective at increasing both size and strength. The adverse effects of water retention and aromatization leading to gynaecomastia are considered to be less pronounced than in long-acting testosterone injections.

5.4.10 SUSTANON 100

As Sustanon 250, but contains

Testosterone propionate	20 mg
Testosterone phenylpropionate	40 mg
Testosterone isocaproate	60 mg

5.4.11 FORMEBOLONE (INJECTABLE)

Alternative name:

Formyldienolone

Proprietary name:

Esiclene (4 mg/2 mL)

Formebolone is a water-based steroid used as a muscle inflammatory. It will inflame a local injection site and cause the muscle to gain size temporarily.

Street information
Esiclene is commonly used in smaller muscles such as biceps, calves or rear deltoids. It is injected directly into the target muscle with an insulin needle, to increase size. Esiclene also adds muscle definition and hardness for the duration of the reaction, which is usually approximately 24 hours. Esiclene has been used over longer periods (weekly injections) in an attempt to stimulate the growth of a specific muscle. The most commonly reported adverse effect is soreness at the site of injection, despite the inclusion of a local anaesthetic in the preparation.

5.4.12 BOLDENONE UNDECANOATE (INJECTABLE)

Alternative name:

Boldenone undecylenate

Veterinary products:

Boldebal-H (50 mg/mL)	Pace (50 mg/mL)
Equipoise (25, 50 mg/mL)	Sybolin (25 mg/mL)
Ganabol (25, 50 mg/mL)	Vebonol (25 mg/mL)

Boldenone undecenoate is an oil-based AS used in veterinary practice. It is highly anabolic and moderately androgenic and is not considered to be toxic to the liver. Drive contains boldenone undecenoate in addition to methandriol dipropionate.

Street information
Equipoise is commonly thought to be effective in producing rapid increases in strength and muscle mass and has also been used for 'cutting' prior to competition. It has a reputation for having low to moderate androgenic properties with little aromatization or water retention. Equipoise also has a reputation for increasing the appetite and for stimulating erythropoiesis.

5.4.13 TESTOSTERONE CYPIONATE (INJECTABLE)

Alternative names:

Testosterone cipionate
Testosterone cyclopentylpropionate

Proprietary names:

Andro-Cyp (100, 200 mg/mL)   Duratest (100, 200 mg/mL)
Depo-Testosterone (50, 100,   Testa-C (200 mg/mL)
   200 mg/mL)   Testex Leo (100, 250 mg/mL)
Depotest (100, 200 mg/mL)

Testosterone cypionate is an ester of testosterone with high anabolic and androgenic properties. It is oil based and therefore long acting. The common side-effects of cypionate are mostly associated with its high androgenic component: testicular atrophy, reduced spermatogenesis and aromatization.

Street information
Testosterone cypionate has a reputation for producing dramatic gains in both size and strength. It is considered to aromatize easily, leading to problems such as gynaecomastia. Large dosages have been associated with causing psychological effects including aggression. Hypertension, acne and premature balding are also commonly reported problems.

5.4.14 TESTOSTERONE ENANTHATE (INJECTABLE)

Alternative names:

Testosterone enantate
Testosterone heptanoate

Proprietary names:

Androtardyl (250 mg/mL)	Primoteston Depot (100, 180 mg/mL)
Delatestryl (200 mg/mL)	Testo-Enant (100, 250 mg/mL)
Durathate (200 mg/mL)	Testosteron-depot (50, 100, 250 mg/mL)
Malogen (100, 200 mg/mL)	Testoviron Depot (100, 250 mg/mL)

Veterinary products:

Testosterona 200 (200 mg/mL)

Street information
Testosterone enanthate is considered to be very similar to testosterone cypionate but less likely to cause water retention.

5.4.15 Testosterone propionate (Injectable)

Alternative name:

Testosteroni propionas

Proprietary names:

Agovirin (25 mg/mL)	Testosterone Streuli (5, 10, 25,
Anrofort Richt (10, 25 mg/mL)	50 mg/mL)
Neo Hombreol (50 mg/mL)	Testoviron (10, 25, 50 mg/mL)
Testex Leo (25 mg/mL)	Testovis (50, 100 mg/mL)
Testosteron (10, 25, 50 mg/mL)	Triolandren (20 mg/mL)
Testosterone Propionicum	Virormone (20, 50, 100 mg/mL)
(10, 25 mg/mL)	

Veterinary products:

Ara-test (25 mg/ml)
Testogan (25 mg/mL)
Testosterona (50 mg/mL)

Testosterone propionate is a fast-acting, short-lasting testosterone ester, with potential adverse effects similar to the enanthate and cypionate. Fifty milligrams of testosterone propionate has been shown to result in elevated testosterone levels for between one and two days. This compares to an elevation in testosterone levels of one to two weeks following the administration of testosterone enanthate.

Street information
Testostosterone propionate has a reputation for being much milder than either the cypionate or enanthate, causing fewer side-effects because of its shorter duration of effect. It is believed to rarely cause hypertension but may aromatize at high dosages.

5.4.16 TESTOSTERONE UNDECANOATE (ORAL)

Proprietary names:

Andriol (40 mg)   Restandol (40 mg)
Androxon (40 mg)   Understor (40 mg)
Pantestone (40 mg)   Virigen (40 mg)

Therapeutic dose:

40–120 mg daily

Testosterone undecanoate is a relatively new AS, having only been available for the past 15 years. It is an oral AS that is not 17-alpha-alkylated and therefore does not have a strong association with liver dysfunction.

Street information
Testosterone undecanoate remains effective in the system for only a few hours and has a particularly short half-life. Many users feel it promotes rapid strength and weight gains. It has a reputation for minimal LH and FSH suppression together with little aromatization. It is considered to virilize easily, making it unpopular with female steroid users.

5.4.17 METHYLTESTOSTERONE (ORAL)

Alternative name:

Methyltestosteronum

Proprietary names:

Afro (25 mg)   Teston (25 mg)
Agovirin (10 mg)   Testormon (10 mg)
Android (5, 10, 25 mg)   Testosteron (5 mg)
Andoral (10 mg)   Testovis (10 mg)
Hormobin (5 mg)   Testred (10 mg)
Mesteron (10 mg)   Virilon (10 mg)
Oreton Methyl (10 mg)

As with other 17-alpha-alkylated AS, methyltestosterone can produce a cholestatic hepatitis with jaundice, especially when given in large doses or for prolonged periods. Methyltestosterone is absorbed from the gastrointestinal tract and from the oral mucosa. It is more resistant to metabolism than testosterone and has a longer half-life.

Street information
Methyltestosterone has a reputation for being highly toxic to the liver, causing hypertension and acne and aromatizing easily. It has also been linked with increased aggression and irritability. Longivol is produced in Spain, and contains vitamins in addition to methyltestosterone.

5.4.18 CLENBUTEROL (ORAL)

Alternative name:

Clenbuterol hydrochloride

Proprietary names:

Broncodil (0.01 mg) Contraspasmina (0.02 mg)
Broncoterol (0.02 mg) Monores (0.01, 0.02 mg)
Cesbron (0.02 mg) Novegam (0.02 mg)
Clembumar (0.02 mg) Prontovent (0.02 mg)
Clenasma (0.02 mg) Spiropent (0.02 mg)
Clenbuter (0.02 mg) Spasmo-Mucosolvan (0.02 mg)
Clenbutol (0.02 mg) Ventolase (0.02 mg)
Contrasmina (0.02 mg)

Also manufactured in aerosol and injection forms but these are rarely available.

Clenbuterol is a direct-acting sympathomimetic agent and is used as a bronchodilator in the management of asthma and obstructive lung disease. It has a considerably longer half-life than other sympathomimetic asthma preparations such as salbutamol. Clenbuterol has been used illicitly in cattle feeds in an attempt to promote weight gain and to increase muscle to lipid mass. Adverse effects typical of sympathomimetic activity have been attributed to such misuse both in farmers in contact with affected cattle and in persons consuming meat products from affected animals. Clenbuterol has become popular as a performance-enhancing drug because of its anabolic/anticatabolic effects. It is also commonly recognized as a fat-burning agent, as it increases the body temperature. Clenbuterol hydrochloride does not have a pharmaceutical licence for use in the UK, but is relatively easily available. The regime of oral administration varies considerably and is dependent on body weight, body temperature, the desired effect and the commonly held belief of rapid receptor downgrade. The most commonly reported side-effects include nervousness, anxiety, tremors, palpitations, tachycardia, headaches and insomnia. These side-effects are commonly considered to be dose related and temporary.

5.4.19 GAMMA-HYDROXYBUTYRATE (ORAL)

Alternative names:

GHB   Liquid Ecstasy
GBH   Sodium Oxybate

Gamma-hydroxybutyrate (GHB) is a naturally occurring metabolite of the amino acid GABA. It has a significant effect on pituitary hormones, specifically GH and prolactin. Athletes use GHB to induce and improve the quality of sleep, and as an aid in the recovery process. Others use GHB as a diuretic or simply to tranquillize themselves. It is known to cause extreme drowsiness, vomiting, muscle cramps and confusion. These adverse effects appear to be dose related, as GHB is available in various strengths, and administering a safe dose is particularly hazardous. Mixed with alcohol, it can cause convulsions and coma.

GHB is a drug developed in the US as a sedative pre-medication to promote sleep before surgery. Because of this the US Food and Drug Administration removed it from the over-the-counter market. GHB is a colourless, odourless liquid with a slightly salty taste and it is sold in small bottles. The long-term effects of repeated GHB use are as yet unknown. GHB is not controlled under the Misuse of Drugs Act but the manufacture and supply are controlled by the Medicines Act.

5.4.20 HUMAN CHORIONIC GONADOTROPHIN (INJECTABLE)

Alternative names:

Choriogonadotrophin   HCG
Chorionic gonadotropin   hCG
Gonadotrophinum chorionicum   Pregnancy-urine hormone

Human chorionic gonadotrophin (hCG) is a hormone produced by the placenta and obtained from the urine of pregnant women. Its effects are predominantly those of the gonadotrophin, luteinizing hormone, and it is used in the treatment of infertile women and in the treatment of delayed puberty in males.

Side-effects that have been reported include headache, tiredness, changes in mood, depression, restlessness, oedema, and pain on injection. There have also been links between hCG and gynaecomastia. hCG should be avoided in individuals for whom androgen-induced fluid retention might be a hazard; for example, those with asthma, epilepsy, migraine, cardiovascular disorders, hypertension and renal disorders. hCG should also be avoided in individuals with disorders that might be exacerbated by androgen release, such as carcinoma of the prostate.

It is relatively common for AS users to use hCG. It has been used to 'kick-start' the natural production of the hormones from the testes that had been suppressed by the higher levels of exogenous steroids. However, it is considered by some that the use of hCG merely carries this effect one more step down the homeostatic-controlled hormonal system. Using hCG not only stimulates testosterone but will also suppress LHRF production from the pituitary. When hCG is stopped there will then be low LHRF leading to low LH levels that in turn will cause suppressed testes function. This means that any benefits from using hCG would be lost in addition to the possibility of the pituitary gland being affected indefinitely.

5.4.21 GROWTH HORMONE (INJECTABLE)

Alternative name:

Somatropin

Human growth hormone (GH) or somatropin is a polypeptide hormone secreted by the anterior pituitary gland. Normal growth in children is dependent upon GH. Growth hormone affects the growth of almost every organ and tissue in the body. It has been shown to cause retention of nitrogen, and an increase in protein synthesis, producing an anabolic effect. Growth hormone also stimulates the mobilization of lipids from adipose tissue and increases their oxidation as a source of energy, thus sparing muscle glycogen. Overproduction of GH before growth is complete can result in gigantism. If it occurs after cessation of growth when the epiphyses have closed, it causes acromegaly. Acromegaly is characterized by an increase in the size of the skull with prominent cheekbones and a protruding jaw and the broadening of the hands and feet. Facial features become coarse as a result of increased growth of subcutaneous tissues.

There is some evidence suggesting a relationship between long-term administration of GH and the development of acute leukaemia, with the incidence of leukaemia in GH-treated patients representing a twofold increase over the expected rate. The use of GH has also been linked to the development of osteoporosis.

A number of deaths from CJD in patients who had received GH extracted from human pituitary glands resulted in the suspension of the distribution of pituitary-derived GH. Synthetic preparations of GH are now available that are free from contamination with the CJD virus. However, because of the long incubation period of this virus, cases of infection are still being reported in patients who had received pituitary-derived GH many years ago.

Athletes using GH to either increase their size and strength or their ultimate height, depending on the maturity of the user, are at risk of developing the clinical syndromes gigantism or acromegaly. Reported side-effects have included skeletal changes, enlargement of internal organs including cardiomegaly, development of diabetes, arthritis, impotence and inflammation and pain at injection sites. One of the most commonly reported adverse effects of GH in athletes is the thickening and coarsening of the skin.

5.4.22 INSULIN-LIKE GROWTH FACTOR 1

Alternative name:

IGF-1

Over the past 18 months, the use of IGF-1 as a performance-enhancing drug by athletes has emerged. This represents a new generation of performance-enhancing drug use by athletes, at a time where possible clinical applications of IGF-1 are only just beginning to emerge. In many ways the use of IGF-1 by athletes is probably more prolific than the use by specialist clinicians. IGF-1 is still considered to be a research tool in medicine, but its traditional function is as a cell culture medium.

IGF-1 is an endogenously produced single-chain polypeptide of 70 amino acids, cross-linked with three disulphide bridges. IGF-1 shows insulin-like properties. It is produced mainly in the liver, under positive control of GH. It circulates in blood as a free form and also bound to binding proteins. Most of the actions of GH, particularly the anabolic actions, are mediated through IGF-1. It has been shown to promote anabolism in humans who have been made catabolic by reduced calorie intake. The main limiting factor of using IGF-1 on its own would appear to be hypoglycaemia; other side-effects include oedema and jaw pain. Recent studies have shown that high nutritional states are necessary for IGF-1 therapy to be maximally effective as an anabolic agent. IGF-1 is especially anabolic for skeletal muscle and it is this property that attracts athletes to its use.

IGF-1 is available as a recombinant form, for example from *Escherichia coli*, and analogues of the original structure are available, with increased efficacy. Manufacturer prices do not match that of the black market. Prices on the street are variable, but in the UK they average around £600 per mg. Counterfeit drugs are a problem for athletes, mainly because they can be contaminated, for example with filler substances or pathogens. As IGF-1 is packaged as a powder for reconstitution in a single glass vial it would be extremely easy to counterfeit.

5.4.23 NALBUPHINE HYDROCHLORIDE (INJECTABLE)

Proprietary name:

Nubain

Nalbuphine hydrochloride is an opioid analgesic with actions and uses similar to morphine. It also has opioid antagonist activity. It is given sub-cutaneously, intramuscularly or intravenously. Nalbuphine hydrochloride is reported to act within 15 minutes of subcutaneous or intramuscular injection or within 2 to 3 minutes of intravenous injection and generally produces analgesia for 3 to 6 hours. It differs from morphine in that its analgesic, sedative and respiratory depressant actions are subject to a 'ceiling' effect and may not increase proportionately with dose. The most frequent side-effects of nubain are drowsiness, sweating, nausea, vomiting, dizziness, vertigo, dry mouth and headache.

Nubain was first used by AS users because of its reputation as an anti-catabolic agent. More recently users have given many diverse explanations for its use including: to enable training with injuries, to mask pain caused by increased weights and to relieve discomfort caused by pre-contest fasting. There have been reports of the development of dependence in individuals using nubain for its perceived performance-enhancing properties.

5.4.24 TAMOXIFEN

Tamoxifen (Nolvadex) is an anti-oestrogenic agent commonly prescribed for the treatment of oestrogen-dependent breast tumours. Tamoxifen achieves this effect by binding to the target receptor sites.

Tamoxifen is available in 10, 20 and 40 mg tablets.

Street information
Tamoxifen is used by AS users to prevent or reduce gynaecomastia, caused by aromatization or when endogenous testosterone levels are suppressed. The effectiveness of Tamoxifen in the prevention of gynaecomastia varies considerably between individuals. Tamoxifen has also been used by steroid users as a dieting aid. It is felt by some that in addition to the prevention of gynaecomastia it may also reduce oedema and prevent female pattern fat distribution.

References

ADVISORY COUNCIL ON THE MISUSE OF DRUGS (ACMD) (1988) *AIDS and Drug Misuse, Part 1.* HMSO, London.

ACMD (1989) *AIDS and Drug Misuse, Part 2.* HMSO, London.

ACMD (1993) *AIDS and Drug Misuse, Update.* HMSO, London.

AIACHE, A. E. (1989) Surgical treatment of gynecomastia in the body builder. *Plastic and Reconstructive Surgery* 83, 61–6.

ALEN, M., REINILIA, M. and VIHKO, R. (1985) Response of serum hormones to androgen administration in power athletes. *Medicine and Science in Sports and Exercise* 17, 354–9.

ALEN, M., RAHKILA, P. and REINILA, M. (1987) Androgenic-anabolic steroid effects on serum thyroid, pituitary and steroid hormones in athletes. *American Journal of Sports Medicine* 15, 357–61.

ANDERSON, W. A. and MCKEAG, D. B. (1985) *The Substance Use and Abuse Habits of College Athletes.* Michigan State University College of Human Medicine. NCAA Athletic Association Council Executive Committee, Drug Education Committee.

ARMSTRONG, D. J. and REILLY, T. (1996) Blood boosting and sport. In *Drugs in Sport* (2nd edn) (ed. D. R. MOTTRAM), pp. 219–34. E & FN Spon, London.

AWIAH, J., BUTT, S. and DORN, N. (1990) The last place I would go. *Druglink* 5(5), 14–15.

BACH, B. R., WARREN, R. F. and WICKIEWICZ, T. L. (1987) Triceps rupture: a case report and literature review. *American Journal of Sports Medicine* 15, 285–9.

BAHR, R. and TJORNHOM, M. (1998) Prevalence of doping in sports: doping control in Norway 1977–1995. *Clinical Journal of Sport Medicine* 8(1), 32–7.

BAHRKE, M., YESALIS, C. and WRIGHT, J. (1990) Psychological and behavioural effects of endogenous testosterone levels and anabolic-androgenic steroids among males: a review. *Sports Medicine* 10, 303–37.

BAHRKE, M., YESALIS, C. and WRIGHT, J. (1996) Psychological and behavioural effects of endogenous testosterone and anabolic-androgenic steroids: an update. *Sports Medicine* 22, 367–90.

BAHRKE, M. S., YESALIS, C. E. and BROWER, K. J. (1998) Anabolic-androgenic steroid abuse and performance-enhancing drugs among adolescents. *Child and Adolescent Psychiatric Clinics of North America* 7(4), 821–38.

BARAHAL, H. S. (1938) Testosterone in male involutional melancholia. *Psychiatric Quarterly* 12, 743–9.

BEARDSWORTH, S. A., KEARNEY, C. E. and PURDIE, D. W. (1999) Prevention of postmenopausal bone loss at lumbar spine and upper femur with tibolone: a two-year randomised controlled trial. *British Journal of Obstetrics and Gynaecology* 106, 678–83.

BEHRENDT, H. and BOFFIN, H. (1977) Myocardial cell lesions caused by an anabolic hormone. *Cell Tissue Research* 181, 423–6.

BELLET, S., KERSHBAUM, A. and ASPE, J. (1965) The effect of caffeine on free fatty acids. *Archives of Internal Medicine* 116, 750–2.

BELLIS, M. (1996) Prevalence and patterns of anabolic steroid use. *The 3rd Annual Conference of The Drugs and Sport Information Service, 2nd July, Liverpool*. Drugs and Sport Information Service, Liverpool.

BEST, D. and MIDGLEY, S. (1999) Assessing HIV risk behavior among users of anabolic steroids in Newcastle upon Tyne. *The Journal of Performance Enhancing Drugs* 2(1), 20–3.

BEST, W. and HENDERSON, D. (1995) Anabolic steroids and the mass media. *Relay* 1(3), 2–4.

BHASIN, S., STORER, T. W., BERMAN, N. *et al.* (1996) The effects of supraphysiologic doses of testosterone on muscle size and strength in normal men. *New England Journal of Medicine* 335, 1–7.

BICKLEMAN, C., FERRIES, L. and EATON, R. P. (1995) Impotence related to anabolic steroid abuse in a body builder. Response to clomiphene citrate. *Western Journal of Medicine* 162, 158–60.

BIRTLES, R. (1998) Trends in anabolic steroid use reported by agency based syringe exchange schemes 1992–1996. *Journal of Performance Enhancing Drugs* 2(2), 22–9.

BLACK, T. and PAPE, A. (1997) The ban on drugs in sports: the solution or the problem? *Journal of Sport and Social Issues* 21(1), 83–92.

BLETHER, S. L., GAINES, S. and WELDON, V. (1984) Comparison of predicted and adult heights in short boys: effect of androgen therapy. *Pediatric Research* 18, 467–9.

BLOUIN, A. and GOLDFIELD, G. (1995) Body image and steroid use in male bodybuilders. *International Journal of Eating Disorders* 18, 159–65.

BOLDING, G., SHERR, L., MAGUIRE, M. and ELFORD, J. (1999) HIV risk behaviours among gay men who use anabolic steroids. *Addiction* 94, 1829–35.

BORG, J. (1973) The effects of smoked marijuana on human cognitive and motor functions. *Psychopharmacology* 29, 159.

BOROWSKY, I. W., HOGAN, M. and IRELAND, M. (1997) Adolescent sexual aggression: risk and protective factors. *Pediatrics* 100(6), E7.

BOWMAN, S. J., TANNON, S., FERNANDO, S., AYODEIL, A. and WEATHERSTONE, R. M. (1989) Anabolic steroids and infarction. *British Medical Journal* 299, 632.

BRADWELL, A. R., DYKES, P. W., COOTE, J. H., FORSTER, P. J. E., MILLES, J. J., CHESNER, I. and RICHARDSON, J. V. (1986) Effect of acetazolamide on exercise performance and muscle mass at high altitude. *Lancet* 1(2), 1001–5.

BRISSON, G. R. (1999) Ergogenic use of growth hormone: a well established habit. *Science* 4(1), 1–6.

BRISTOW, C. (1992) Detective Inspector, Metropolitan Police. Personal communication.

British National Formulary (2001) The British Medical Association and the Royal Pharmaceutical Society of Great Britain, London.

BRODIE, D. A. and TOWSE, S. (1999) The effects of creatine supplementation during weight training. *Journal of Performance Enhancing Drugs* 2(3), 18–25.

BRONSON, F. (1996) Effects of prolonged exposure to anabolic steroids on the behaviour of male and female mice. *Pharmacology and Biochemistry of Behaviour* 53, 49–55.

BRONSON, F. H. and MATHERNE, C. M. (1997) Exposure to anabolic-androgenic steroids shortens life span of male rats. *Medicine and Science in Sports and Exercise* 29, 615–19.

BROWER, K. J. (1992) Addictive potential of anabolic steroids. *Psychiatric Annals* 22, 30–4.

BROWER, K. J. (1993) Assessment and treatment of anabolic steroid withdrawal. In *Anabolic Steroids in Sport and Exercise* (ed. C. E. YESALIS), pp. 231–52. Human Kinetics, Champaign, IL.

BROWER, K. J., BLOW, F., YOUNG, J. and HILL, E. M. (1991) Symptoms and correlates of anabolic-androgenic steroid dependence. *British Journal of Addiction* 86, 759–68.

BROWER, K. J., BLOW, F. C. and HILL, E. M. (1994) Risk factors for the anabolic-androgenic steroid use in men. *Journal of Psychiatric Research* 28, 369–80.

BROWN, L. S., PHILLIPS, R. Y., BROWN, C. L., KNOWLAN, D., CASTLE, L. and MOYER, J. (1994) HIV/AIDS policies and sports: The National Football League. *Medicine and Science in Sports and Exercise* 26(4), 403–7.

Brown University Digest of Addiction Theory and Application (1994) Steroid use associated with other drug use, aggression. *The Brown University Digest of Addiction Theory and Application* 13(4), 10.

BRUHN, P. and MAAGE, N. (1975) Intellectual and neuropsychological functions in young men with heavy and long-term patterns of drug abuse. *American Journal of Psychiatry* 132(4), 397–401.

BRYDEN, A. A., ROTHWELL, P. J. and O'REILLY, P. H. (1995) Anabolic steroid abuse and renal cell carcinoma. *Lancet* 346, 1306–7.

BUCKLEY, W., YESALIS, C. E., FRIEDL, K. E., ANDERSON, W. A., STREIT, A. L. and WRIGHT, J. E. (1988) Estimated prevalence of anabolic steroid use among male high school seniors. *Journal of the American Medical Association* 260(23), 3441–5.

BUTENANDT, A. and TSCHERNING, K. (1934a) Uber Androsteron, ein krystallisiertes Mannliches Sexualhormon I. Isoliereng und Reindarstellung aus Mannerharn. *Zeitschrift fuer Physiologische Chemie* 229, 167–84.

BUTENANDT, A. and TSCHERNING, K. (1934b) Uber Androsteron ein Krystallisiertes Sexualhormon II. *Zeitschrift fuer Physiologische Chemie* 229, 185–91.

CABASSO, A. (1994) Peliosis hepatitis in a young adult body builder. *Medicine and Science in Sports and Exercise* 26, 2–4.

CABLE, N. T. and TODD, L. (1996) Coronary heart disease risk factors in bodybuilders using anabolic steroids. *Journal of Performance Enhancing Drugs* 1, 25–8.

CALABRESE, L. H., KLEINER, S. M., BARNA, B. P., SKIBINSKI, C. I., KIRKENDALL, D. T., LAHITA, R. G. and LOMARDO, J. A. (1989) The effects of anabolic steroids and strength training on the human immune response. *Medicine and Science in Sports and Exercise* 21, 386–92.

CANTWELL, J. D. and ROSE, F. D. (1986) Cocaine and cardiovascular events. *The Physician and Sportsmedicine* 14(11), 77–82.

CASHMORE, E. (1990) *Making Sense of Sport*. Routledge, London.

CHOI, P. and POPE, H. G., JR (1994) Violence toward women and illicit androgenic-anabolic steroid use. *Annals of Clinical Psychiatry* 6(1), 21–5.

CHOI, P., PARROTT, A. and COWAN, D. (1990) High-dose anabolic steroids in strength athletes: effects upon hostility and aggression. *Human Psychopharmacology* 5, 349–56.

CLARKE, J. (1999) Anabolic steroids – a growing problem. Network Northwest. *Healthwise Liverpool*, edition no. 10, Liverpool.

CLARKSON, P. M. (1996) Nutrition for improved sports performance. *Current Issues On Ergogenic Aids* 21, 393–401.

CLEMMONS, D. R. (1993) Use of growth hormone and IGF1. *Hormone Research* 40(1–3), 62–7.

COHEN, J. C. and HICKERMAN, R. (1987) Insulin resistance and diminished glucose tolerance in power lifters ingesting anabolic steroids. *Journal of Clinical Endocrinology and Metabolism* 64, 960–3.

COHEN, J. C., MIEKE FABER, W., SPINNLER-BENADE, A. J. and NOAKES, T. D. (1986) Altered serum lipoprotein profiles in male and female power lifters ingesting anabolic steroids. *The Physician and Sportsmedicine* 14(6), 131–6.

COLLINS, P. and COTTERILL, J. A. (1995) Gymnasium acne. *Clinical and Experimental Dermatology* 20, 509.

CONLEE, R. K. (1991) Amphetamine, caffeine and cocaine. In *Perspectives in Exercise Science and Sports Medicine 4* (eds D. R. LAMB and M. H. WILLIAMS), pp. 285–328. Brown & Benchmark, New York.

COOPER, C. (1994) Factors undermining the success of prevention and harm reduction strategies for anabolic-androgenic steroid abuse. In *State of the Art in Higher Education* (eds D. ADEY, P. STEYN, N. HERMAN *et al.*). University of South Africa, Pretoria.

COOPER, C. J., NOAKES, T. D., DUNNE, T., LAMBERT, M. I. and ROCHFORD, K. (1996) A high prevalence of abnormal personality traits in chronic users of anabolic-androgenic steroids. *British Journal of Sports Medicine* 30, 246–50.

COPELAND, J., PETERS, R. and DILLON, P. (2000) Anabolic-androgenic steroid use: disorders among a sample of Australian competitive and recreational users. *Drug and Alcohol Dependence* 60(1), 91–6.

CORRADO, D., THIENE, G., NAVA, A., ROSSINI, L. and PENNELLI, N. (1990) Sudden death in young competitive athletes: clinicopathologic correlations in 22 cases. *American Journal of Medicine* 89, 588–96.

CORRIGAN, B. (1996) Anabolic steroids and the mind. *Medical Journal of Australia* 165, 222–6.

Council of Europe, Strasbourg, 8 July 1998. *Use of Anabolic Steroids and other Doping Substances Outside Competitive Sport.* Literature review and European key informant survey.

Council of Europe, Press Release, Brussels, 30 November 2001. Fight against doping in sport: the EU takes the lead. http://europa.eu.int/comm/sport/index

COWART, V. S. (1988) Human growth hormone: the latest ergogenic aid? *The Physician and Sportsmedicine* 16(3), 175–85.

CREAGH, T. M., RUBIN, A. and EVANS, D. J. (1988) Hepatic tumours induced by anabolic steroids in an athlete. *Journal of Clinical Pathology* 41, 441–3.

CRIST, D. M., PEAKE, G. T., EGAN, P. A. *et al.* (1988) Body composition response to exogenous GH during training in highly conditioned adults. *Journal of Applied Physiology* 65, 579–84.

CSAKY, T. Z. (1972) Doping. *Journal of Sports Medicine and Physical Fitness* 12, 117–23.

CURRY, L. A. and WAGMAN, D. F. (1999) Qualitative description of the prevalence and use of anabolic androgenic steroids by United States powerlifters. *Perceptual and Motor Skills* 88, 224–33.

DALBY, J. (1992) Brief anabolic steroid use and sustained behavioural reaction, *American Journal of Psychiatry* 149, 271–2.

DANZINGER, L. and BLANK, H. R. (1942) Androgen therapy of agitated depressions in the male. *Medical Annals of the District of Columbia* 11(5), 181–3.

DAVIDOFF, E. and GOODSTONE, G. L. (1942) Use of testosterone propionate in treatment of involutional psychosis in the male. *Archives of Neurology and Psychiatry* 48, 811–17.

DAWSON, R. T. (2001) Drugs in sport – the role of the physician. *Journal of Endocrinology* 170, 55–61.

DELBEKE, F. T., DESMET, N. and DEBACKERE, M. (1995) The abuse of doping agents in competing body builders in Flanders (1988–1993). *International Journal of Sports Medicine* 16(1), 66–70.

DE MERODE, A. (1988) The development, objectives and activities of the IOC Medical Commission. In *The Olympic Book of Sports Medicine* (eds A. DIRIX, H. G. KNUTTGREN and K. TITTEL), pp. 3–12. Blackwell Scientific Publishers, Oxford.

DEMLING, R. H. (1999) Comparison of the anabolic effect and complications of human growth hormone and the testosterone analog, oxandrolone, after severe burn injury. *Burns* 25(3), 215–21.

DE PICCOLI, B. (1991) Anabolic steroid use in bodybuilders: an ethnographic study of left ventricle morphology and function. *International Journal of Sports Medicine* 12, 1–3.

DERY, D. (1984) *Problem Definition in Policy Analysis*. University of Kansas Press, Lawrence, Kansas.

DEYSSIG, R. and WEISSEL, M. (1993) Ingestion of androgenic-anabolic steroids induces mild thyroidal impairment in male body builders. *Journal of Clinical Endocrinology and Metabolism* 76, 1069–71.

DICKERMAN, R. D., McCONATHY, W. J., SCHALLER, F. and ZACHARIAH, N. Y. (1996) Cardiovascular complications and anabolic steroids. *European Heart Journal* 17, 1912.

DICKERMAN, R. D., SCHALLER, F., ZACHARIAH, N. Y. and McCONATHY, W. J. (1997) Left ventricular size and function in elite bodybuilders using anabolic steroids. *Clinical Journal of Sport Medicine* 7(2), 90–3.

DICKERMAN, R. D., SCHALLER, F. and McCONATHY, W. J. (1998) Left ventricular wall thickening does occur in elite power athletes with or without anabolic steroid use. *Cardiology* 90(2), 145–8.

DICKERMAN, R. D., PERTUSI, R. M., ZACHARIAH, N. Y., DUFOUR, D. R. and McCONATHY, W. J. (1999) Anabolic steroid-induced hepatotoxicity: is it overstated? *Clinical Journal of Sport Medicine* 9(1), 34–9.

DICKMAN, S. (1991) East Germany: science in the disservice of the state; a secret East German program to perfect steroid drugs for athletes was a full fledged scientific endeavour. *Science* 254(5028), 26–8.

DOBS, A. S. (1999) Is there a role for androgenic anabolic steroids in medical practice? *Journal of the American Medical Association*, 281(14), 1326–7.

DOHERTY, M. (1996) Caffeine: effects on short-term, high-intensity exercise. *Journal of Performance Enhancing Drugs* 1, 135–43.

DONIKE, M. and STRATMANN, D. (1974) Temperature programmed gas chromato-graphic analysis of nitrogen containing drugs. Reproducibility screening procedure for volatile drugs at the 20th Olympic Games, Munich, 1972. *Chromatographia* 7(4), 182–9.

DONOHOE, T. and JOHNSON, N. (1986) *Drug Abuse in Sport*. Blackwell, Oxford.

DUBIN, C. L. (1990) *Commission of Inquiry into the Use of Drugs and Banned Practices Intended to Increase Athletic Performance*. Canadian Government Publishing Centre, Ottawa, Canada.

DUCHAINE, D. (1989) *The Underground Steroid Handbook* (2nd edn). HLR Technical Books, Venice, CA.

DUDA, M. (1986a) Cocaine deaths may increase drug tests. *The Physician and Sportsmedicine* 14(8), 37.

DUDA, M. (1986b) Female athletes: targets for drug abuse. *The Physician and Sportsmedicine* 14(6), 142–6.

DUFF, R. and HONG, L. (1984) Self images of women bodybuilders. *Sociology of Sport* 1(4), 374–80.

DURANT, R. H., RICKERT, V. I., ASHWORTH, C. S., NEWMAN, C. and SLAVENS, G. (1993) Use of multiple drugs among adolescents who use anabolic steroids. *The New England Journal of Medicine* 328(13), 922–7.

DURANT, R. H., RICKERT, V. I., ASHWORTH, C. S., NEWMAN, C. and SLAVENS, G. (1997) Adolescent anabolic-androgenic steroid use, multiple drug use, and high school sports participation. *Pediatric Exercise Science* 9, 150–8.

EICHNER, E. R. (1997) Ergogenic aids: what athletes are using and why. *The Physician and Sportsmedicine* 25(4), 70–83.

ELKIN, S. L., BRADY, S. and WILLIAMS, I. P. (1997) Bodybuilders find it easy to obtain insulin to help them in training. *British Medical Journal* 314, 1280.

ELLINGROD, V. L., PERRY, P. J., YATES, W. R., MacINDOE, J. H., WATSON, J. H., ARNDT, S. and HOLMAN, T. L. (1997) *The American Journal of Drug and Alcohol Abuse* 23(4), 623–36.

ELLIOT, D. and GOLDBERG, L. (1996) Intervention and prevention of steroid use in adolescents. *American Journal of Sports Medicine* 24, S46–7.

EVANS, N. A. (1997) Local complications of self administered anabolic steroid injections. *British Journal of Sports Medicine* 31, 207–8.

EVANS, N. A., BOWREY, D. J. and NEWMAN, G. R. (1998) Ultrastructural analysis of ruptured tendon from anabolic steroid users. *Injury* 29, 769–73.

EVELY, R. S., TRIGER, D. R., MILNES, J. P., LOW-BEER, T. S. and WILLIAMS, R. (1987) Severe cholestasis associated with stanozolol. *British Medical Journal* 294, 612–13.

FAIGENBAUM, A. D., ZAICHKOWSKY, L. D., GARDNER, D. E. and MICHELI, L. J. (1998) Anabolic steroid use by male and female middle school students. *Pediatrics* 101(5), E6.

FENICHEL, G., PRESTRONK, A., FLORENCE, J., ROBINSON, V. and HEMELT, V. (1997) A beneficial effect of oxandrolone in the treatment of Duchenne muscular dystrophy: a pilot study. *Neurology* 48, 1225–6.

FERENCHICK, G. S. (1990) Are androgenic steroids thrombogenic? *New England Journal of Medicine* 322, 476.

FERENCHICK, G. S. and ADELMAN, S. (1992) Myocardial infarction associated with anabolic steroid use in a previously healthy 37-year-old weight lifter. *American Heart Journal* 124, 507–8.

FERENCHICK, G. S., KIRLIN, P. and POTTS, R. (1991) Steroids and cardiomyopathy: how strong a connection. *Physician and Sports Medicine* 19, 107–8.

FERRANDEZ, M. D., DE LA FUENTE, M., FERNANDEZ, E. and MANSO, R. (1996) Anabolic steroids and lymphocyte function in sedentary and exercise-trained rats. *Journal of Steroid Biochemistry and Biological Biology* 59, 225–32.

FERREIRA, I. M., VERRESCHI, I. T., NERY, L. E. *et al.* (1998) The influence of 6 months of oral anabolic steroids on body mass and respiratory muscles in undernourished COPD patients. *Chest* 114, 19–28.

FINLAY, M. and PLECKET, H. (1976) *The Olympic Games: The First Hundred Years.* Chatto & Windus, London.

FISCHMAN, M. W. (1987) Cocaine and amphetamines. In *Psychopharmacology: The Third Generation of Progress* (ed. H. Y. MELTZER), p. 1543. Raven Press, New York.

FOWLER, L. J., SMITH, S. S., SNIDER, T. and SCHULTZ, M. R. (1996) Apocrine metaplasia in gynecomastia by fine needle aspiration as a possible indicator of anabolic steroid use. A report of two cases. *Acta Cytologica* 40, 734–8.

FRANCIS, C. (1990) *Speed Trap.* Grafton, Collins, London.

FRANKLE, M. A., EICHBERG, R. and ZACHARIAH, S. B. (1988) Anabolic-androgenic steroids and a stroke in an athlete. *Archives of Physical Medicine and Rehabilitation* 69, 632–3.

FREED, D., BANKS, A. J. and LONGSON, D. (1972) Anabolic steroids in athletes. *British Medical Journal* 3, 761.

FREED, D. L. J., BANKS, A. J., LONGSON, D. and BURLEY, D. M. (1975) Anabolic steroids in athletics: cross over double blind trial on weight lifters. *British Medical Journal* 2, 471–3.

FREEDSON, P., CHANGE, B., KATCH, F., KROLL, J., RIPPE, J., ALPERT, J. and BYRNES, W. (1984) Intra-arterial blood pressure during free weight and hydraulic resistance exercise. *Medicine and Science in Sports Medicine* 16, 131.

FRIEDL, K. E. (1993) Effects of anabolic steroids on physical health. In *Anabolic Steroids in Sport and Exercise* (ed. C. E. YESALIS), pp. 107–48. Human Kinetics, Champaign, IL.

FRIEDL, K. E. and YESALIS, C. E. (1989) Self treatment of gynecomastia in body builders who use anabolic steroids. *The Physician and Sports Medicine* 17, 67–79.

FRUEHAN, A. E. and FRAWLEY, T. F. (1963) Current status of anabolic steroids. *Journal of the American Medical Association* 184(7), 527–32.

FUSSELL, S. (1991) *Muscle: Confessions of an Unlikely Bodybuilder.* Scribners, London.

GALLAGHER, T. F. and KOCH, F. C. (1934) The testicular hormone. *Journal of Biological Chemistry* 84, 495–500.

GEORGE, A. (1996a) The anabolic steroids and peptide hormones. In *Drugs in Sport* (2nd edn) (ed. D. R. MOTTRAM), pp. 173–218. E & FN Spon, London.

GEORGE, A. (1996b) Central nervous system stimulants. In *Drugs in Sport* (2nd edn) (ed. D. R. MOTTRAM), pp. 86–112. E & FN Spon, London.

GERRITSMA, E. J., BROCAAR, M. P., HAKKESTEEGT, M. M. and BIRKENHAGER, J. C. (1994) Virilization of the voice in post-menopausal women due to the anabolic steroid nandrolone decanoate (Decadurabolin). The effects of medication for one year. *Clinical Otolarynology* 19, 79–84.

GILBERT, B. (1969) Drugs in sport: part 2. Something extra on the ball. *Sports Illustrated* 30–5.

GILL, G. V. (1998) Anabolic steroid induced hypogonadism treated with human chorionic gonadotropin. *Postgraduate Medical Journal* 74(867), 45–6.

GLASS, A. R. and Vigersky, R. A. (1980) Resensitization of testosterone production in men after human chorionic gonadotrophin-induced desensitization. *Journal of Clinical Endocrinology and Metabolism* 51, 1395–400.

GLAZER, G. (1991) Atherogenic effects of anabolic steroids on serum lipid levels: a literature review. *Archives of Internal Medicine* 151, 1925–33.

GLAZER, G. and SUCHMAN, A. L. (1994) Lack of demonstrated effect of nandrolone on serum lipids. *Metabolism* 43, 204–10.

GOLD, M. S. and ESTROFF, T. W. (1984) The comprehensive evaluation of cocaine and opiate abusers. In *Handbook of Psychiatric Diagnostic Procedures* (vol. 2) (eds R. C. W. HALL and R. BERESFORD), p. 213. Spectrum Publications, Englewood Cliffs.

GOLDMAN, B. (1984) *Death in the Locker Room*. Elite Sports Medicine Publications Ltd, Chicago.

GOLDMAN, B. and KLATZ, R. (1992) *Death in the Locker Room* II. Elite Sports Medicine Publications Ltd, Chicago.

GOLDMAN, S. F. and MARKHAM, M. J. (1942) Clinical use of testosterone in the male climacteric. *Journal of Clinical Endocrinology* 2, 237–42.

GOLDSTEIN, D., DOBBS, T., KRULL, B. and PLUMB, V. J. (1998) Clenbuterol and anabolic steroids – a previously unreported cause of myocardial infarction with normal coronary angiograms. *Southern Medical Journal* 91(8), 780–4.

GREEN, D. J., CABLE, N. T., RANKIN, J. M., FOX, C. and TAYLOR, R. R. (1993) Anabolic steroids and vascular responses. *Lancet* 342, 863.

GREENBERG, S., GEORGE, W. R., KADOWITZ, P. J. and WILSON, W. R. (1974) Androgen-induced enhancement of vascular reactivity. *Canadian Journal of Physiology and Pharmacology* 52, 12–22.

GREENWAY, P. and GREENWAY, M. (1997) General practitioner knowledge of prohibited substances in sport. *British Journal of Sports Medicine* 31(2), 129–31.

GRIVETTI, L. E. and APPLEGATE, E. A. (1997) From Olympia to Atlanta: a cultural–historical perspective on diet and athletic training. *The Journal of Nutrition* 127(5), 860–8s.

GROSSMAN, C. J. (1985) Interactions between the gonadal steroids and the immune system. *Science* 227, 257–61.

GRUBER, A. J. and POPE, H. G. (2000) Psychiatric and medical effects of anabolic-androgenic steroid use on women. *Psychotherapy and Psychosomatics* 69(1), 19–26.

GURAKAR, A., CARACENI, P., FAGIUOLI, S. and VAN THEIK, D. H. (1994) Androgenic/anabolic steroid-induced intrahepatic cholestasis: a review with four additional case reports. *Journal of the Oklahoma State Medical Association* 87, 399–404.

GUYTON, A. G. (1986) *Textbook of Medical Physiology* (7th edn). W. B. Saunders, Philadelphia.

HAKKINEN, K. and ALEN, M. (1989) Training volume, androgen use and serum creatine kinase activity. *British Journal of Sports Medicine* 23, 188–9.

HAMILTON, J. B. (1937) Treatment of sexual underdevelopment with synthetic male hormone substance. *Endocrinology* 21, 649–54.

HANDELSMAN, D. J. and GUPTA, L. (1997) Prevalence and risk factors for anabolic-androgenic steroid abuse in Australian high school students. *International Journal of Andrology* 20(3), 159–64.

HART, M. (1993) *Steroids: The Layman's Guide*. Mick Hart Training Systems, UK.

HAUPT, H. A. (1993) Anabolic steroids and growth hormone. *American Journal of Sports Medicine* 21, 468–74.

HAUPT, H. A. and ROVERE, G. D. (1984) Anabolic steroids: a review of the literature. *American Journal of Sports Medicine* 12, 469–84.

HAYNES, R. C. and MURAD, F. (1985) Adrenocorticosteroids and their synthetic analogs: inhibitors of adrenocortical steroid biosynthesis. In *Goodman and Gilman's*

The Pharmacological Basis of Therapeutics (7th edn) (eds A. G. GILMAN *et al.*), p. 1459. Macmillan, New York.

HEBBELINCK, M. (1959) The effects of a moderate dose of alcohol on a series of functions of physical performance in man. *Archives Internationales de Pharmacodynamie et de Therapie* 120, 402.

HEBBELINCK, M. (1963) The effects of a small dose of ethyl alcohol on certain basic components of human physical performance. *Archives Internationales de Pharmacodynamie et de Therapie* 143, 247.

HEIKKALA, J. (1993) Modernity, morality and the logic of competing. *International Review for the Sociology of Sport* 28, 355–69.

HEINONEN, O. J. (1996) Carnitine and physical exercise. *Sports Medicine* 22, 109–32.

HENRION, R., MANDELBROT, L. and DELFIEU, D. (1992) Contamination par le VIH a la suite d'injections d'anabolisants. *La Presse Medicale* 21, 218.

HERVEY, G. R., HUTCHINSON, I., KNIBBS, A. V., BURKINSHAW, L., JONES, P. R. M., NORGAN, N. G. and LEVELL, M. J. (1976) Anabolic effects of methandienone in men undergoing athletic training. *Lancet* 2, 699–702.

HEYDENREICH, G. (1989) Testosterone and anabolic steroids and acute fulminans. *Archives of Dermatology* 125, 571–2.

HICKSON, R. C., BALL, K. L. and FALDUTO, M. T. (1989) Adverse effects of anabolic steroids. *Medical Toxicology in Adverse Drug Experience* 4, 254–71.

HOBERMAN, J. (1990) The transformation of East German sport. *Journal of Sport History* 17(1), 62–8.

HOBERMAN, J. M. and YESALIS, C. E. (1995) The history of synthetic testosterone. *Scientific American* February, 60–5.

HOLLISTER, L. (1986) Health aspects of cannabis. *Pharmacological Reviews* 38, 1.

HOLMA, P. (1977a) Effect of an anabolic steroid (Methandienone) on central and peripheral blood flow in well-trained male athletes. *Annals of Clinical Research* 9, 215–21.

HOLMA, P. K. (1977b) Effects of an anabolic steroid (Methandienone) on spermatogenesis. *Contraception* 15, 157–62.

HOSKINS, R. G. (1941) *Endocrinology, the Glands and their Function.* Norton, New York.

HUGHES, T. K., FULEP, E., JUELICH, T., SMITH, E. M. and STANTON, G. J. (1995) Modulation of immune responses by anabolic steroids. *International Journal of Immunopharmacology* 17, 857–63.

HUIZENGA, R. (1994) *You're Okay It's Just a Bruise.* St Martin's Press, New York.

JAFFE, J. H. (1985) Opioid dependence. In *Comprehensive Textbook of Psychiatry IV* (4th edn) (eds H. I. KAPLAN and B. J. SADDOCK), p. 1008. Williams & Wilkins, Baltimore.

JAFFE, J. H. and MARTIN, W. R. (1985) Opioid analgesics and antagonists. In *Goodman and Gilman's The Pharmacological Basis of Therapeutics* (7th edn) (eds A. G. GILMAN *et al.*), p. 491. Macmillan, New York.

JENNINGS, A. (1996) *The New Lords of the Rings.* Pocket Books, London.

JIN, B., TURNER, L., WALTERS, W. A. and HANDLESON, D. J. (1996) Androgen or estrogen effects on human prostate. *Journal of Clinical Endocrinology and Metabolism* 81, 4290–5.

JOHNSON, L. C. and O'SHEA, J. P. (1968) Anabolic steroids: effects on strength and development. *Science* 164, 957–9.

JOHNSON, M. D. (1990) Anabolic steroid use in adolescent athletes. *Pediatric Clinics of North America* 37, 1111–23.

JOHNSON, M. D., JAY, S., SHOUP, B. and RICKERT, V. I. (1989) Anabolic steroid use by male adolescents. *Pediatrics* 83(6), 921–4.

KANE, M. J. (1988) Media coverage of the female athlete, before, during and after title IX: Sports Illustrated revisited. *Journal of Sport Management* 2(2), 87–99.

KANE, M. J. and SNYDER, E. (1989) Sport typing: the social containment of women. *Arena Review* 13(2), 77–96.

KANTOR, M. A., BIANCHINI, A., BERNIER, D., SADY, S. P. and THOMPSON, P. D. (1985) Androgens reduce HDL2-cholesterol and increase hepatic triglyceride lipase activity. *Medicine and Science in Sports and Exercise* 17, 462–5.

KASHKIN, K. B. and KLEBER, H. D. (1989) Hooked on hormones? An anabolic steroid hypothesis. *Journal of the American Medical Journal* 262, 3166–70.

KATZ, F. H. and ROPER, E. F. (1977) Testosterone effect on renin system in rats. *Proceedings of the Society for Experimental Biology and Medicine* 155, 330–3.

KENDRICK, C. (1999) *Seduced by Steroids.* Family Education Network. http://familyeducation.com/fec/articlepage

KENNEDY, M. C. and LAWRENCE, C. (1993) Anabolic steroid abuse and cardiac death. *Medical Journal of Australia* 158, 346–8.

KERSEY, R. D. (1996) Anabolic-androgenic steroid use among California Community College student athletes. *Journal of Athletic Training* 31, 237–41.

KHANKHANIAN, N. K., HAMMERS, Y. A. and KOWALSKI, P. (1992) Exuberant local tissue reaction to intramuscular injection of nandrolone decanoate (Deca-Durabolin) – a steroid compound in a sesame oil base – mimicking soft tissue malignant tumours: a case report and review of the literature. *Military Medicine* 157, 670–4.

KHANTZIAN, E. J. and McKENNA, G. J. (1979) Acute toxic and withdrawal reactions associated with drug use and abuse. *Annals of Internal Medicine* 90, 361.

KIBBLE, M. W. and ROSS, M. B. (1987) Adverse effects of anabolic steroids in athletes. *Clinical Pharmacy* 6, 686–92.

KICMAN, A. T. and COWAN, D. A. (1992) Peptide hormones and sport: misuse and detection. *British Medical Bulletin* 48(3), 496–517.

KICMAN, A. T., BROOKS, R. V. and COWAN, D. A. (1991) Human chorionic gonadotrophin and sport. *British Journal of Sports Medicine* 25(2), 73–9.

KINDLUNDH, A. M., ISACSON, D. G., BERGLUND, L. and NYBERG, F. (1998) Doping among high school students in Uppsala, Sweden: a presentation of the attitudes, distribution, side effects, and extent of use. *Scandinavian Journal of Social Medicine* 26(1), 71–4.

KLAVA, A., SUPER, P., ALDRIGE, M., HORNER, J. and GUILLOU, P. (1994) Body builder's liver. *Journal of the Royal Society of Medicine* 87, 43–4.

KLEIN, A. (1984) Pumping iron: crisis and contradiction in bodybuilding. *Sociology of Sport* 3, 112–33.

KLEINER, S. M., CALABRESE, L. H., FIEDLER, K. M., NAITO, H. K. and SKIBINSK, C. I. (1989) Dietary influences on cardiovascular risk in anabolic steroid using over non-using bodybuilders. *Journal of the American College of Nutrition* 8, 109–19.

KOCHAKIAN, C. D. (1935) Effect of male hormone on protein metabolism of castrate dogs. *Proceedings for the Society for Experimental Biology and Medicine* 32, 1064–5.

KOCHAKIAN, C. D. (1975) Definition of androgens and protein anabolic steroids. *Pharmacology and Therapeutics B* 1(2), 149–77.

KOCHAKIAN, C. D. (1976) Metabolic effects of anabolic-androgenic steroids in experimental animals. In *Handbook of Experimental Pharmacology: vol. 43. Anabolic-Androgenic Steroids* (ed. C. D. KOCHAKIAN), pp. 5–44. Springer-Verlag, Berlin.

KOCHAKIAN, C. D. (1993a) Anabolic-androgenic steroids: a historical perspective and definition. In *Anabolic Steroids in Sports and Exercise* (2nd edn) (ed. C. E. YESALIS), pp. 3–33. Human Kinetics, Champaign, IL.

KOCHAKIAN, C. D. (1993b) History, chemistry and pharmacodynamics of anabolic-androgenic steroids. *Wiener Medizinische Wochenschrift* 143(14–15), 359–63.

KOCHAKIAN, C. D. and ENDAHL, B. R. (1959) Changes in body weight of normal and castrated rats by different doses of testosterone propionate. *Proceedings of the Society for Experimental Biology and Medicine* 100, 520–2.

KOCHAKIAN, C. D. and MURLIN, J. (1935) The effect of male hormone on the protein and energy metabolism of castratee dogs. *Journal of Nutrition* 10, 437–59.

KOLLER, W. C. and BIARY, N. (1984) Effects of alcohol on tremors: comparison with propanolol. *Neurology* 34, 221.

KOMOROSKI, E. M. and RICKERT, V. I. (1992) Adolescent body image and attitudes to anabolic steroid use. *American Journal of Diseases of Children* 146(7), 823–8.

KORKIA, P. (1997) Anabolic steroid use: a survey of general practitioners in the South of England. (Abstract) *The Proceedings of the 2nd European Congress of Sport and Exercise Science.* Copenhagen.

KORKIA, P. and STIMSON, G. V. (1993) *Anabolic Steroid Use in Great Britain: An Exploratory Investigation.* A report for the Department of Health, the Welsh Office and the Chief Scientist Office, Scottish Home and Health Department. The Centre For Research on Drugs and Health Behaviour, London.

KORKIA, P. and STIMSON, G. V. (1997) Indications of prevalence, practice and effects of anabolic steroid use in Great Britain. *International Journal of Sports Medicine* 18(7), 557–62.

KORKIA, P., LENEHAN, P. and McVEIGH, J. (1996) Non-medical use of androgens among women. *The Journal of Performance Enhancing Drugs* 1(2), 71–6.

KORTE, T., PYKALAINEN, J. and SEPPALA, T. (1998) Drug abuse of Finnish male prisoners in 1995. *Forensic Science International* 97(2–3), 171–83.

KOURI, E. M., LUKAS, S. E., POPE, H. G., JR and OLIVA, P. S. (1995) Increased aggressive responding in male volunteers following the administration of gradually increasing doses of testosterone cypionate. *Drug and Alcohol Dependency* 40(1), 73–9.

KOURI, E. M., POPE, H. G. and OLIVA, P. S. (1996) Changes in lipoprotein-lipid levels in normal men following administration of increasing doses of testosterone cypionate. *Clinical Journal of Sports Medicine* 6, 152–7.

KRAMHOFT, M. and SOLGAARD, S. (1986) Spontaneous rupture of the extensor pollius longus tendon after anabolic steroids. *Journal of Hand Surgery* 11, 87.

DE KRUIF, P. (1945) *The Male Hormone.* Harcourt, Brace & Company, New York.

KUIPERS, H., WIJNEN, J. A. G., HARTGENS, F. and WILLEMS, S. M. M. (1991) Influence of anabolic steroids on body composition, blood pressure, lipid profile and liver functions in body builders. *International Journal of Sports Medicine* 12, 413–18.

LAJARIN, F., ZARAGOZA, R., TOVAR, I. and MARTINEZ-HERNANDEZ, P. (1996) Evolution of serum lipids in two male bodybuilders using anabolic steroids. *Clinical Chemistry* 42, 970–2.

LAKE, C. R. and QUIRK, R. S. (1984) CNS stimulants and the look-alike drugs. *Psychiatric Clinics of North America* 7, 689–701.

LAMB, D. R. (1984) Anabolic steroids in athletics: how well do they work and how dangerous are they? *American Journal of Sports Medicine* 12, 31–8.

LAMBERT, M. I., TITLESTAD, S. D. and SCWELLNUS, M. P. (1998) Prevalence of androgenic-anabolic steroid use in adolescents in two regions of South Africa. *South African Medical Journal* 88(7), 876–80.

LANGSTON, J. W. and LANGSTON, E. B. (1986) Neurological consequences of drug abuse. In *Diseases of the Nervous System: Clinical Neurobiology* (eds A. K. ASBURY, G. M. MCKHANN and W. I. MCDONALD), p. 1333. W. B. Saunders, Philadelphia.

LAROCHE, G. P. (1990) Steroid anabolic drugs and arterial complications in an athlete – a case history. *Angiology* 41, 964–9.

LASETER, J. T. and RUSSELL, J. A. (1991) Anabolic steroid-induced tendon pathology: a review of the literature. *Medicine and Science in Sports and Exercise* 23, 1–3.

LAURE, P. (1998) Doping in amateur adult athletes aged 15 or over. *Journal of Performance Enhancing Drugs* 2(2), 16–19.

LENAWAY, D., GUILIFOILE, B. and REBCHOOK, A. (1992) Multiple HIV risk behaviours among injection-steroid users. *AIDS and Public Policy Journal* 7, 182–6.

LENDERS, J. W. M., DEMACKER, P. N. M., VOS, J. A., JANSEN, P. L. M., HOITSMA, A. J., VAN'T LAAR, A. and THIEN, T. (1988) Deleterious effects of anabolic steroids on serum lipoproteins, blood pressure and liver function in amateur body builders. *Journal of Sports Medicine* 9, 19–23.

LENEHAN, P. (1997) *Anabolic Steroids: A Guide for Professionals*, Chapters 2 and 6. Drugs and Sport Information Service, Liverpool.

LENEHAN, P. and MCVEIGH, J. (1994) HIV and steroid use. *Relay* 1(2), 19–20.

LENEHAN, P. and MCVEIGH, J. (1996) *Anabolic steroid use in Liverpool*. Liverpool, The Drugs and Sport Information Service, Liverpool.

LENEHAN, P., BELLIS, M. and MCVEIGH, J. (1996) Anabolic steroid use in the north west of England. *Journal of Performance Enhancing Drugs* 1, 57–70.

LENSKYJ, H. (1986) *Out of Bounds: Women, Sport and Sexuality*. Women's Press, Toronto, Ontario.

LINDHOLM, C., HIRSCHBERG, A. L., CARLSTROM, K. and VON SCHOULTZ, B. (1995) Altered adrenal steroid metabolism underlying hypercortisolism in female endurance athletes. *Fertility and Sterility* 63, 1190–4.

LINDSTROM, M., NILSSON, A., KATZMAN, P. et al. (1990) Use of anabolic-androgenic steroids among bodybuilders – frequency and attitudes. *Journal of Internal Medicine* 227, 407–11.

LLOYD, F. H., POWELL, P. and MURDOCH, A. P. (1996) Anabolic steroid abuse by body builders and male subfertility. *British Medical Journal* 313, 100–1.

LOMBARDO, J. A. (1986) Stimulants and athletic performance (part 1 of 2): amphetamines and caffeine. *The Physician and Sportsmedicine* 14(11), 128–40.

LONGHURST, J. C., KELLY, A. R., CONYEA, W. J. and MITCHELL, J. M. (1980) Echocardiographic left ventricular masses in distance runners and weight lifters. *Journal of Applied Physiology* 48, 154–62.

LOPES, J. M., JARDIN, J., AUBIER, M. et al. (1983) Effect of caffeine on skeletal muscle function before and after fatigue. *Journal of Applied Physiology* 54, 1303–5.

LUBELL, A. (1989) Does steroid abuse cause or excuse violence. *The Physician and Sportsmedicine* 17(2), 176–86.

LUESCHEN, G. (1993) Doping in sport: the social structure of a deviant subculture. *Sports Science Review* 2(1), 92–126.

LUKAS, S. E. (1996) CNS effects and abuse liability of anabolic-androgenic steroids. *Annual Reviews of Pharmacology and Toxicology* 36, 333–57.

LUKE, J. L., FAREB, A., VIRMANI, R. and SAMPLE, R. H. B. (1990) Sudden cardiac death during exercise in a weight lifter using anabolic androgenic steroids: pathological and toxicological findings. *Journal of Forensic Science* 35, 1441–7.

LUMIA, A., THORNER, K. and McGINNIS, M. (1994) Effects of chronically high doses of the anabolic androgenic steroid, testosterone on intermale aggression and sexual behaviour in male rats. *Physiology and Behaviour* 55, 331–5.

MALARKEY, W. B., STRAUSS, R. H., LEIZMEN, D. J., LIGGETT, M. T. and DEMERS, L. M. (1991) Endocrine effects in women weight lifters self administering testosterone and anabolic steroids. *American Journal of Obstetrics* 165, 1385–90.

MANDELL, A. J. (1979) The Sunday syndrome: a unique pattern of amphetamine abuse indigenous to American professional football. *Clinical Toxicology* 15, 225–32.

MARON, B. J., ROBERTS, W. C., McALLISTER, H. A., ROSING, D. R. and EPSTEIN, S. E. (1980) Sudden death in young athletes. *Circulation* 62, 218–29.

MAYCOCK, B. (1999) Factors contributing to androgenic steroid related violence. *Journal of Performance Enhancing Drugs* 2(3), 4–15.

McBRIDE, A. J., WILLIAMSON, K. and PETERSON, T. (1996) Three cases of nalbuphine hydrochloride dependence associated with anabolic steroid use. *British Journal of Sports Medicine* 30, 69–70.

McCAUGHAN, G. W., BILOUS, M. J. and GALLAGHER, N. D. (1985) Long term survival with tumour regression in androgen-induced liver tumours. *Cancer* 56, 2622–6.

McGEE, L. C. (1927) The effect of injection of a lipoid fraction of bull testicle in capons. *Proceedings of the Institute of Medicine* 6, 242.

McKILLOP, G., TODD, I. C. and BALLANTYNE, D. (1986) Increased left ventricular mass in a body builder using anabolic steroids. *British Journal of Sports Medicine* 20, 151–2.

McKILLOP, G., BALLANTYNE, F. C., BORLAND, W. and BALLANTYNE, D. (1989) Acute metabolic effects of exercise in body builders using anabolic steroids. *British Journal of Sports Medicine* 23, 186–7.

McNUTT, R. A., FERENCHICK, G. S., KIRLIN, P. C. and HAMLIN, N. J. (1988) Acute myocardial infarction in a 22-year-old world class weight lifter using anabolic steroids. *American Journal of Cardiology* 62, 164.

McVEIGH, J. and LENEHAN, P. (1994) Counterfeits and fakes: a growing problem. *Relay* 1(1), 8–9.

McVEIGH, J. and LENEHAN, P. (1995) Gym owners opinions on performance enhancing drugs. *Relay* 1(3), 19–20.

MELCHERT, R. B. and WELDER, A. A. (1995) Cardiovascular effects of androgenic-anabolic steroids. *Medicine and Science in Sport and Exercise* 27, 1252–62.

MELCHERT, R. B., HERRON, T. J. and WELDER, A. A. (1992) The effect of anabolic-androgenic steroids on primary myocardial cell cultures. *Medicine and Science in Sport and Exercise* 24, 206–12.

MELIA, P. (1994) Is sport a healthy place for children? *Relay* (2), 10–12.

MELIA, P., PIPE, A. and GREENBERG, L. (1996) The use of anabolic-androgenic steroids by Canadian students. *Clinical Journal of Sport Medicine* 6(1), 9–14.

MENAPACE, F. J., HAMMER, W. J., RITZER, T. F., KESSLER, K. M., WARNER, H. F., SPANN, J. F. and BORE, A. A. (1982) Left ventricular size in competitive weight lifters: an echocardiographic study. *Medicine and Science in Sports and Exercise* 14, 72–5.

MENARD, C. S., HEBERT, T. J., DOHANICH, G. P. and HARLAN, R. E. (1995) Androgenic-anabolic steroids modify beta-endorphin immunoreactivity in the rat brain. *Brain Research* 669, 255–62.

MENDENHALL, C. L., GROSSMAN, C. J. and ROSELLE, G. A. (1990) Anabolic steroid effects on immune function: differences between analogues. *Journal of Steroid Biochemical and Molecular Biology* 37, 71–6.

MENDENHALL, C. L., MORITZ, T. E., ROSELLE, G. A. *et al.* (1995) Protein energy malnutrition in severe alcoholic hepatitis: diagnosis and response to treatment. *Journal of Parenteral and Enteral Nutrition* 19, 258–65.

METROPOLITAN BOROUGH OF SEFTON (1998) *Young People in The Metropolitan Borough of Sefton*. Schools Health Education Unit, Sefton.

MEWIS, C., SPYRIDOPOULOS, I., KUHLKAMP, V. and SEIPEL, L. (1996) Manifestation of severe coronary heart disease after anabolic drug abuse. *Clinical Cardiology* 19, 153–5.

MIDDLEMAN, A. B., FAULKNER, A. H., WOODS, E. R., EMANS, S. J. and DURANT, R. H. (1995) High-risk behaviors among high school students in Massachusetts who use anabolic steroids. *Pediatrics* 96, 268–72.

MIDGLEY, S. J., HEATHER, N., BEST, D., HENDERSON, D., MCCARTHY, S. and DAVIES, J. B. (2000) Risk behaviours for HIV and hepatitis infection among anabolic-androgenic steroid users. *AIDS Care* 12(2), 163–70.

MILLAR, A. P. (1994) Licit steroid use – hope for the future. *British Journal of Sports Medicine* 28, 79–83.

MILLAR, A. P. (1996) Anabolic steroids – a personal pilgrimage. *Journal of Performance Enhancing Drugs* 1(1), 4–9.

MILLER, W. S., DACKIS, C. A. and GOLD, M. S. (1987) The relationship of addiction, tolerance and dependence to alcohol and drugs: a neurochemical approach. *Journal of Substance Abuse Treatment* 4, 197.

MINKIN, D., MEYER, M. and VAN HAAREN, F. (1993) Behavioural effects of longterm administration of an anabolic steroid in intact and castrated male Wistar rats. *Pharmacology and Biochemistry of Behaviour* 44, 959–63.

MOCHIZUKI, R. M. and RICHTER, K. J. (1988) Cardiomyopathy and cerebrovascular accident associated with anabolic-androgenic steroid use. *The Physician and Sportsmedicine* 16, 109–14.

MONTINE, T. J. and GAEDE, J. T. (1992) Massive pulmonary embolus and anabolic steroid abuse. *Journal of the American Medical Association* 267, 2328–9.

MORRISON, C. L. (1994) Anabolic steroid users identified by needle and syringe exchange contact. *Drug and Alcohol Dependence* 36, 153–6.

MORRISON, C. L. (1996) Cocaine misuse in anabolic steroid users. *Journal of Performance Enhancing Drugs* 1, 10–15.

MOSS, H. B., PANZAK, G. L. and TARTER, R. E. (1993) Sexual functioning of male anabolic steroid abusers. *Archives of Sexual Behaviour* 22, 1–12.

MOTTRAM, D. R. (1996) What is a drug? In *Drugs in Sport* (2nd edn) (ed. D. R. MOTTRAM), pp. 1–17. E & FN Spon, London.

MYERS, J. and EARNEST, M. (1984) Generalized seizures and cocaine abuse. *Neurology* 34, 675.

NAGHII, M. R. (1999) The significance of dietary boron, with particular reference to athletes. *Nutrition and Health* 13(1), 31–7.

NAKAO, J., CHANGE, W. C., MUROTA, S. I. and ORIMO, H. (1981) Testosterone inhibits prostacyclin production by rat aortic smooth muscle cells in culture. *Atherosclerosis* 39, 203–9.

NAKATA, S. (1997) Prostate cancer associated with long-term intake of patent medicine containing methyltestosterone: a case report. *Hinyokika Kiyo* 43, 791–3.

NEMECHEK, P. M. (1991) Anabolic steroid users: another potential risk group for HIV infection. *New England Journal of Medicine* 325, 357.

NEWERLA, G. J. (1943) The history of the discovery and isolation of the male hormone. *New England Journal of Medicine* 228, 39–47.

NIEMINEN, M. S., RAMO, M. P., VIITASALO, M., HEIKKILA, P., KARJALAINEN, J., MANTYSAARI, M. and HEIKKILA, J. (1996) Serious cardiovascular side effects of large doses of anabolic steroids in weight lifters. *European Heart Journal* 17, 1576–83.

NILSSON, S. (1995) Androgenic anabolic steroid use among male adolescents in Falkenberg. *European Journal of Clinical Pharmacology* 48(1), 9–11.

NOCELLI, L., KAMBER, M., FRANCOIS, Y., GMEL, G. and MARTI, B. (1998) Discordant perception of doping in elite versus recreational sport in Switzerland. *Clinical Journal of Sport Medicine* 8(3), 195–200.

NODEN, M. (1994) Dying to win. *Sports Illustrated* 81(6), 52–60.

NUNES, E. V. and ROSECAN, J. S. (1987) Human neurobiology of cocaine. In *Cocaine Abuse: New Directions in Treatment and Research* (eds H. I. SPITZ and J. S. ROSECAN), p. 48. Brunner/Mazel, New York.

NUTTER, J. (1997) Middle school students' attitudes and use of anabolic steroids. *Journal of Strength and Conditioning Research* 11, 35–9.

O'CONNOR, S. (1995) Why do bodybuilders take anabolic steroids? *Relay* 2(1), 4–5.

OVERLY, W. L., DANKOFF, J. A., WANG, B. K. and SINGH, U. D. (1984) Androgens and hepatocellular carcinoma in an athlete. *Annals of Internal Medicine* 100, 158–9.

PAPADAKIS, M. A., GRADY, D., BLACK, D. *et al.* (1996) Growth hormone replacement in healthy older men improves body composition but not functional ability. *Annals of Internal Medicine* 124(8), 708–16.

PARKES, A. S. (1985) *Off Beat Biologist: The Autobiography of AS Parkes*. The Galton Foundation, Cambridge, England.

PARROTT, A., CHOI, P. and DAVIES, M. (1994) Anabolic steroid use by amateur athletes: effects upon psychological mood states. *Journal of Sports Medicine and Physical Fitness* 34, 292–8.

PARRY, D. A. (1996) Insulin-like growth factor 1 (IGF 1): a new generation of performance enhancement by athletes. *Journal of Performance Enhancing Drugs* 1, 48–51.

PARSSINEN, M., KUJALA, U., VARTIAINEN, E., SARNA, S. and SEPPALA, T. (2000) Increased premature mortality of competitive powerlifters suspected to have used anabolic agents. *International Journal of Sports Medicine* 21(3), 225–7.

PASTERNAK, G. (1982) High and low affinity opioid binding sites: relationship to mu and delta sites. *Life Sciences* 31, 1303.

PEARSON, A. C., SCHIFF, M., ROSEK, D., LABOVITZ, A. J. and WILLIAMS, G. A. (1986) Left ventricular diastolic function in weight lifters. *American Journal of Cardiology* 58, 1254–9.

PEDERSEN, B. K. and BRUUNSGAARD, H. (1995) How physical exercise influences the establishment of infections. *Sports Medicine* 19, 393–400.

PENA, N. (1991) Lethal injection: cycling's new wonder drug can kill you. *Bicycling* April, 80–1.

PENTEL, P. (1984) Toxicity of over-the-counter stimulants. *Journal of the American Medical Association* 252, 1898–903.

PERRY, H. (1995) Counterfeit-fake anabolic steroids and hazards of their use. *Relay* 1(4), 9–12.

PERRY, H. and HUGHES, G. W. (1992) A case of affective disorder associated with the misuse of 'anabolic steroids'. *British Journal of Sports Medicine* 26(4), 219–20.

PERRY, H., WRIGHT, D. and LITTLEPAGE, B. N. C. (1992) Dying to be big: a review of anabolic steroid use. *British Journal of Sports Medicine* 26, 259–61.

PERRY, P. J., ANDERSON, K. H. and YATES, W. R. (1990a) Illicit anabolic steroid use in athletes. *American Journal of Sports Medicine* 18, 422–8.

PERRY, P., YATES, W. and ANDERSON, K. (1990b) Psychiatric symptoms associated with anabolic steroids: a controlled, retrospective study. *Annals of Clinical Psychiatry* 2, 11–17.

PETERS, M. and MARSHALL, J. (1993) Educational policy analysis and the politics of interpretation. *Evaluation Review* 17(3), 310–30.

PETERSON, G. E. and FAHEY, T. D. (1984) HDL-C in five elite athletes using anabolic-androgenic steroids. *The Physician and Sports Medicine* 12, 120–30.

PETTINE, K. A. (1991) Association of anabolic steroids and avascular necrosis of femoral heads. *American Journal of Sports Medicine* 19, 96–8.

PHILIPS, W. N. (1991) *Anabolic Reference Guide* (6th issue). Mile High Publishing, Colorado.

PLAUS, W. J. and HERMAN, G. (1991) The surgical management of superficial infections caused by atypical mycobacteria. *Surgery* 110, 99–103.

POPE, H. G., JR. and KATZ, D. L. (1988) Affective and psychotic symptoms associated with anabolic steroid use. *American Journal of Psychiatry* 145, 487–90.

POPE, H. G., JR. and KATZ, D. L. (1990) Homicide and near-homicide by anabolic steroid users. *Journal of Clinical Psychiatry* 51(1), 28–31.

POPE, H. G. and KATZ, D. L. (1992) Psychiatric effects of anabolic steroids. *Psychiatric Annals* 22, 24–9.

POPE, H. G. and KATZ, D. (1994) Psychiatric and medical effects of anabolic-androgenic steroid use. *Archives of General Psychiatry* 51, 373–82.

POPE, H. G., JR, KOURI, E. M., POWELL, K. F., CAMPBELL, C. and KATZ, D. L. (1996) Anabolic-androgenic steroid use among 133 prisoners. *American Journal of Psychiatry* 153(10), 1369.

POPE, H. G., JR, KOURI, E. M. and HUDSON, J. I. (2000) Effects of supraphysiologic doses of testosterone on mood and aggression in normal men: a randomised controlled trial. *Archives of General Psychiatry* 57(2), 133–40.

PORCERELLI, J. H. and SANDLER, B. A. (1995) Narcissism and empathy in steroid users. *American Journal of Psychiatry* 152(11), 1672–4.

PRATHER, I. D., BROWN, D. E., NORTH, P. and WILSON, J. (1995) Clenbutarol: a substitute for anabolic steroids? *Medicine and Science in Sports and Exercise* 27, 1118–21.

RAMOTAR, J. E. (1990) Cyclists' deaths linked to erythropoietin? *The Physician and Sportsmedicine* 18(8), 48–9.

REILLY, T. (1996) Alcohol, anti-anxiety drugs and sport. In *Drugs in Sport* (2nd edn) (ed. D. R. MOTTRAM), pp. 144–72. E & FN Spon, London.

REJESKI, W., GREGG, E., KAPLAN, J. R. and MANUCK, S. B. (1990) Anabolic steroids: effects on social behaviour and baseline heart rate. *Health and Psychology* 9, 774–91.

RENAUD, A. M. and CORMIER, Y. (1986) Acute effects of marijuana on maximal exercise performance. *Medicine and Science in Sports and Exercise* 18, 685–9.

REYES, R. J., ZICCHI, S., HAMED, H., CHAUDARY, M. A. and FENTIMAN, I. S. (1995) *British Journal of Clinical Practice* 49, 177–9.

RING, M. E. and BUTMAN, S. M. (1986) Cocaine and premature myocardial infarction. *Drug Therapy* September, 117.

RITSCH, M. and MUSSHOFF, F. (2000) Dangers and risks of black market anabolic steroid abuse in sports – gas chromatography–mass spectrometry analyses. *Sportverletz Sportschaden* 14(1), 1–11.

ROCHFORT, D. A. and COBB, R. W. (1994) *The Politics of Problem Definition*. University Press of Kansas, Lawrence, Kansas.

ROCKHOLD, R. W. (1993) Cardiovascular toxicity of anabolic steroids. *Annual Review of Pharmacology and Toxicology* 32, 497–520.

ROGERS, P. J., RICHARDSON, N. J. and DERNONCOURT, C. (1995) Caffeine use: is there a net benefit for mood and psychomotor performance? *Neuropsychobiology* 31, 195–9.

ROSENFELD, R. G., NORTHCRAFT, G. B. and HENTZ, R. L. (1982) A prospective, randomised study of testosterone treatment of constitutional delay of growth and development in male adolescents. *Pediatrics* 68, 681–7.

ROSENKRANTZ, P., VOGEL, S., BEE, H., BROVERMAN, I. and BROVERMAN, D. M. (1968) Sex role stereotypes and self concepts in college students. *Journal of Consulting and Clinical Psychology* 32, 287–95.

RUSSELL-JONES, D. L. and UMPLEBY, M. (1996) Protein anabolic action of insulin, growth hormone and insulin-like growth factor 1. *European Journal of Endocrinology* 135, 631–42.

RUZICKA, L., GOLDBERG, M. W., MEYER, J., BRUNIGGER, H. and EICHENBURG, E. (1934) Zur Kenntnis der Sexualhormon II. Uber die Synthesis des Testikelhormons (Androsteron) und Stereoisomers desselben durch Abbau Hydrieter Sterine. *Helvetica Chimica Acta* 17, 1395–406.

RYAN, A. J. (1978) Anabolic steroids: the myth dies hard. *Physician and Sports Medicine* March, 3.

RYAN, A. J. (1981) Anabolic steroids are fools gold. *Federation Proceedings* 40, 2682–8.

SALKE, R. C., ROWLAND, T. W. and BURKE, E. J. (1985) Left ventricular size and function in body builders using anabolic steroids. *Medicine and Science in Sports and Exercise* 17, 701–4.

SALVA, P. S. and BACON, G. E. (1991) Anabolic steroids: interest among parents and nonathletes. *Southern Medical Journal* 84(5), 552–6.

SCARPINO, V., ARRIGO, A., BENZI, G., GARATTINI, S., LA VECCHIA, C., BERNARDI, L. R., SILVESTRINI, G. and TUCCIMEI, G. (1990) Evaluation and prevalence of 'doping' among Italian athletes. *Lancet* 336(8722), 1048–50.

SCHALLY, A. V. and COMARU-SCHALLY, A. M. (1987) Male contraception involving testosterone supplementation: possible increased risks of prostate cancer? *Lancet* i, 448–9.

SCHOLS, A. M., SOERTERS, P. B., MOSTERT, R., PLUMYERS, R. J. and WOUTERS, E. F. (1995) Physiologic effects of nutritional support and anabolic steroids in patients with chromic obstructive pulmonary disease: a placebo controlled randomised trial. *American Journal of Respiratory and Critical Care Medicine* 152(4), 1268–74.

SCHROFF, J. M. (1992) Pumped up (teen use of steroids). *U.S. News and World Report* 112(21), 54–60.

SCHROR, K., MORINELLI, T. A., MASUDA, A., MATSUDA, K., MATHUR, R. S. and HALUSHKA, P. V. (1994) Testosterone treatment enhances thromboxane A2 mimetic induced coronary artery vasoconstriction in guinea pigs. *European Journal of Clinical Investigations* 24(suppl. 1), 50–2.

SCHULTE, H., HALL, M. and BOYER, M. (1993) Domestic violence associated with anabolic steroid abuse. *American Journal of Psychiatry* 150, 348.

SCOTT, M. J. and SCOTT, M. J. (1989) HIV infection associated with injections of anabolic steroids. *Journal of the American Medical Association* 262, 207–8.

SCOTT, M. J. and SCOTT, A. M. (1992) Effects of anabolic-androgenic steroids on the pilosebaceous unit. *Cutis* 50(2), 113–16.

SCOTT, M. J., SCOTT, M. J. and SCOTT, A. M. (1994) Linear keloids resulting from abuse of anabolic androgenic steroid drugs. *Cutis* 53, 41–3.

SHAPIRO, H. (1992) Adjusting to steroid users. The challenges of attracting and adjusting to a new drug agency client group. *Druglink* Sept/Oct, 16–17.

SHEPHERD, R. J., KILLINGER, D. and FRIED, T. (1977) Responses to sustained use of anabolic steroid. *British Journal of Sports Medicine* 11, 170–3.

SKLAREK, H., MANTOVANI, R., ERENS, E., HEISLER, D., NIEDERMAN, M. and FEIN, A. (1984) AIDS in a bodybuilder using anabolic steroids. *New England Journal of Medicine* 311, 1701.

SMITH, D. (1968) The acute and chronic toxicity of marijuana. *Psychedelic Drugs* 2, 347.

SOE, K. L., SOE, M. and GLUUD, C. (1992) Liver pathology associated with the use of anabolic-androgenic steroids. *Liver* 12, 73–9.

SOETENS, E., DE-MEIRLEIR, K. and HUETING, J. E. (1995) No influence of ACTH on maximal performance. *Psychopharmacology, Berlin* 118, 260–6.

STANLEY, A. and WARD, M. (1994) Anabolic steroids – the drugs that give and take away manhood: a case with an unusual sign. *Medicine, Science, and the Law* 34, 82–3.

STIMSON, G. V. (2000) *The Unhealthy State of British Drugs Policy*, presented at the Methadone Alliance Conference, 22 March, London.

STRAUSS, R. H. (1984) Drugs in sport. In *Sports Medicine* (ed. R. H. STRAUSS), pp. 281–491. W. B. Saunders, Philadelphia.

STRAUSS, R. H. (1987) Anabolic steroids. In *Drugs and Performance in Sports* (ed. R. H. STRAUSS), pp. 62–3. W. B. Saunders, Philadelphia.

STRAUSS, R. H., WRIGHT, J. E. and FINERMAN, G. A. M. (1982) Anabolic steroid use and health status among forty-two weight trained male athletes. *Medicine and Science in Sports and Exercise* 14, 119.

STRAUSS, R. H., LIGGETT, M. and LANESE, R. (1985) Steroid use and perceived effects in ten weight trained women athletes. *Journal of the American Medical Association* 253, 2871–3.

STRAWFORD, A., BARBIERI, T., VAN LOAN, M. *et al.* (1999) Resistance exercise and supraphysiologic androgen therapy in eugonadal men with HIV related weight loss: a randomised controlled trial. *Journal of the American Medical Association* 281, 1282–90.

SU, S. T., PAGLIARO, M., SCHMIDT, P. J., PICKAR, D., WOLKOWITZ, O. and RUBINOW, D. R. (1993) Neuropsychiatric effects of anabolic steroids in male normal volunteers. *Journal of the American Medical Association* 269(21), 2760–5.

SULLIVAN, M. L., MARTINEZ, C. M. and GALLAGHER, E. J. (1999) Atrial fibrillation and anabolic steroids. *The Journal of Emergency Medicine* 21, 412–18.

TANNER, S. M., MILLER, D. W. and ALONGI, C. (1995) Anabolic steroid use by adolescents: prevalence, motives, and knowledge of risks. *Clinical Journal of Sport Medicine* 5(2), 108–15.

TAYLOR, W. N. (1991) *Macho Medicine*. McFarland & Company Inc., Jefferson, North Carolina.

TENNANT, F., BLACK, D. L. and VOR, R. O. (1988) Anabolic steroid dependence with opioid-type features. *New England Journal of Medicine* 262, 578.

TERUEL, J. L., AGUILERA, A., AVILA, C. and ORTUNO, J. (1996) Effects of androgen therapy on prostatic markers in hemodialyzed patients. *Scandinavian Journal of Urology and Nephrology* 30, 129–31.

The United Kingdom Anti-Drugs Co-ordinator (1998/1999) *First Annual Report and National Plan.* Cabinet Office, Central Office of Information, London.

THEIN, L. A., THEIN, J. M. and LANDRY, G. L. (1995) Ergogenic aids. *Physical Therapy* 75, 426–39.

THILIBIN, I., RUNESON, B. and RAJS, J. (1999) Anabolic steroids and suicide. *Annals of Clinical Psychiatry* 11, 223–31.

THIBILIN, I., LINDQUIST, O. and RAJS, J. (2000) Cause and manner of death among users of anabolic androgenic steroids. *Journal of Forensic Science* 45, 16–23.

THOMPSON, C. H., KEMP, G. J., SANDERSON, A. L., DIXON, R. M., STYLES, P., TAYLOR, D. J. and RADDA, G. K. (1996) Effect of creatine on aerobic and anaerobic metabolism in skeletal muscle in swimmers. *British Journal of Sports Medicine* 30, 222–5.

THOMPSON, P. D., SADANIANTZ, A., CULLINANE, E. M., BODZIONY, K. S., CATLIN, D. H., TOREK-BOTH, G. and DOUGLAS, P. S. (1992) Left ventricular function is not impaired in weight lifters who use anabolic steroids. *Journal of the American College of Cardiologists* 19, 278–82.

TODD, T. (1987) Anabolic steroids: the gremlins of sport. *Journal of Sport History* 14, 87–107.

TRICKER, R., O'NEILL, M. R. and COOK, D. (1989) The incidence of anabolic steroid use among competitive bodybuilders. *Journal of Drug Education* 19(4), 313–25.

TUREK, P. J., WILLIAMS, R. H., GILBAUGH, J. H. and LIPSHULTZ, L. I. (1995) The reversibility of anabolic steroid-induced azoospermia. *The Journal of Urology* 153, 1628–30.

VAN HANDEL, P. J. (1980) Effects of caffeine on physical performance. *Journal of Operational Research* February, 56–7.

VARRIALE, P., MIRZAI-TEHRANE, M. and SEDIGHI, A. (1999) Acute myocardial infarction associated with anabolic steroids in a young HIV-infected patient. *Pharmacotherapy* 19(7), 881–4.

VERROKEN, M. (1996) Drug use and abuse in sport. In *Drugs in Sport* (2nd edn) (ed. D. R. MOTTRAM), pp. 18–55. E & FN Spon, London.

VERROKEN, M. and MOTTRAM, D. R. (1996) Doping control in sport. In *Drugs in Sport* (2nd edn) (ed. D. R. MOTTRAM), pp. 235–63. E & FN Spon, London.

Voy, R. (1991) *Drugs, Sport and Politics*. Human Kinetics, Champaign, IL.

Wade, N. (1972) Anabolic steroids: doctors denounce them, but athletes aren't listening. *Science* 176, 1399–403.

Wadler, G. I. and Hainline, B. (1989) *Drugs and the Athlete*. FA Davis, Philadelphia.

Wallechinsky, D. (1996) *The Complete Book of the Olympics*. Aurum Press, London.

Wallgren, H. and Barry, H. (1970) *Actions of Alcohol* (vols 1 and 2). Elsevier, New York.

Walsh, D. (1998) Drugs push sport into moral crisis. *The Sunday Times*, 2nd August.

Weil, A. (1925) The history of internal secretions. *M. Life* 32, 73–97.

Weiner, N. (1985) Norepinephrine, epinephrine and the sympathomimetic amines. In *Goodman and Gilman's The Pharmacological Basis of Therapeutics* (7th edn) (eds A. G. Gilman *et al.*), p. 145. Macmillan, New York.

Weiss, B. and Laties, V. G. (1962) Enhancement of human performance by caffeine and the amphetamines. *Pharmacological Reviews* 14, 1–36.

Weiss, R. J. (1986) Recurrent myocardial infarction caused by cocaine abuse. *American Heart Journal* 111, 793.

Wemyss-Holden, S. A., Hamdy, F. C. and Hastie, K. J. (1994) Steroid abuse in athletes, prostatic enlargement and bladder outflow obstruction – is there a relationship? *British Journal of Urology* 74, 476–8.

Westaby, D., Ogle, S. J., Paradinas, F. J., Randell, J. B. and Murray-Lyon, I. M. (1977) Liver damage from long-term methyltestosterone. *Lancet* 1, 261–3.

Whittle, J. (1998) Tour trips through drugs haze. *The Times*, 27th July.

Williams, M. (1969) Effect of selected doses of alcohol on fatigue parameters of the forearm flexor muscles. *Research Quarterly* 40, 832.

Williams, M. H. (1997) *The Ergogenics Edge*, pp. 115–278. Human Kinetics, Champaign, IL.

Williams, M. H. and Branch, J. D. (1998) Creatine supplementation and exercise performance: an update. *Journal of the American College of Nutrition* 17(3), 216–34.

Williamson, D. (1994) What are the psychological effects of anabolic steroid use? *Relay* 1(1), 2–3.

Williamson, D. J. (1993) Anabolic steroid use among students at a British college of technology. *British Journal of Sports Medicine* 27, 200–1.

Williamson, D. J. and Young, A. H. (1992) Psychiatric effects of androgenic and anabolic-androgenic steroid abuse in men: a brief review of the literature. *Journal of Psychopharmacology* 6, 20–6.

Wilson, D. M., Kei, J. and Hintz, R. L. (1988) Effects of testosterone therapy for pubertal delay. *American Journal of Diseases in Children* 142, 96–9.

Wilstein, S. (1998) *Supplement, McGwire linked throughout the 'Net*. http://www.s-t.com/daily/12-98/12-09-98/d05sp165.htm.

Work, J. A. (1991) Are java junkies poor sports? *The Physician and Sportsmedicine* 19(1), 83–8.

World Health Organization (WHO) Task Force on Methods for the Regulation of Male Fertility (1990) Contraceptive efficacy of testosterone-induced azoospermia and oligozoospermia in normal men. *Lancet* 336, 955–9.

Wright, J. M. (1978) *Anabolic Steroids and Sports*. Sports Science Consultants, Natrick, MA.

YARASHEKI, K. E., CAMBELL, J. A., SMITH, K. *et al.* (1992) Effect of growth hormone and resistance exercise on muscle growth in young men. *American Journal of Physiology* 262(1), E261–7.

YARASHEKI, K. E., ZACHWIEJA, J. J., ANGELOPOULOS, T. J. *et al.* (1993) Short-term growth hormone treatment does not increase muscle protein synthesis in experienced weight lifters. *Journal of Applied Physiology* 74(6), 3037–76.

YATES, W. R., PERRY, P. J., MACINDOE, J., HOLMAN, T. and ELLINGROD, V. (1999) Psychosexual effects of three doses of testosterone cycling in men. *Biological Psychiatry* 45(3), 254–60.

YEN, S. and JAFFE, R. (1978) *Reproductive Endocrinology.* W. B. Saunders, Philadelphia.

YESALIS, C. E. (ed.) (1993) *Anabolic Steroids in Sport and Exercise.* Human Kinetics, Champaign, IL.

YESALIS, C. E. and COWART, V. (1998) *The Steroids Game.* Human Kinetics, Champaign, IL.

YESALIS, C. E., COURSON, S. P. and WRIGHT, J. (1993a) History of anabolic steroid use in sport and exercise. In *Anabolic Steroids in Sport and Exercise* (ed. C. E. YESALIS), pp. 35–47. Human Kinetics, Champaign, IL.

YESALIS, C. E., KENNEDY, N. J., KOPSTEIN, A. N. and BAHRKE, M. S. (1993b) Anabolic-androgenic steroid use in the United States. *Journal of the American Medical Association* 270(10), 1217–21.

YESALIS, C. E., BARSUKIEWICZ, C. K., KOPSTEIN, A. N. and BAHRKE, M. S. (1997) Trends in anabolic-androgenic steroid use among adolescents. *Archives of Pediatrics and Adolescent Medicine* 151(12), 1197–206.

ZORNETZER, S. F., WALKER, D. W., HUNTER, B. E. and ABRAHAM, W. C. (1982) Neurophysiological changes produced by alcohol. In *Biomedical Processes and Consequences of Alcohol Use*, p. 95. US Department of Health and Human Services. US Government Printing Office, Washington, DC.

ZULIANI, U., BERNARDINI, B., CATAPANO, A., CAMPANA, M., CERIOLI, G. and SPATTINI, M. (1988) Effect of anabolic steroids, testosterone and HGH on blood lipids and echocardiographic parameters in body builders. *International Journal of Sports Medicine* 10, 6266.

Index

AS refers to anabolic steroids.

abscess formation 47, 48
accidental death 56
acetazolamide 81
acne fulminans 44
acne vulgaris 43–4, 102, 103
acromegaly 84–5, 98, 113, 114
addiction 54, 57
  amphetamines 75
  caffeine 77
adolescents 10, 11
  medical aspects of use 50–1
  prevalence of use 12–15
  females 16, 49
adrenaline 75, 89
adrenocorticotrophic hormone (ACTH) 83–4
advertising 16
aggression 23, 24, 41, 53, 54
  amphetamines 25, 62
  cocaine 25
  driving behaviour 51–2
  elevated feeling 55, 56
  females 50, 52
  inclination to use AS 56
  testosterone/testosterone complexes 52
  violent crime precursor 55
  see also sexual aggression
aging
  males 26
  reversal 63
AIDS 47
  see also HIV infection
alanine transaminase 36

alcohol 61, 62, 70
  cocaine combination 97
  consumption 62
  IOC restrictions 87–8
alkaline phosphate 36
5-alpha reduction 55
amenorrhoea 50
American College of Sports Medicine (ACSM) 8, 65
American football 62, 73
American Medical Association (AMA) 25
γ-aminobutyric acid (GABA) receptors 55
amotivational syndrome 89
amphetamines 47, 62
  adverse effects 76
  aggression 25
  American football 73
  athletes 76
  AS combination 93
  concomitant use 96
  IOC banned list 75–6
  IOC testing 67
amputation 34
anabolic-androgenic steroids 2, 80
  high androgenic 94
anabolic changes 2
anabolic steroids
  commercially available 8
  detection tests 10
  efficacy 93
  ergogenic uses 7–9
  functional uses 66
  prevalence of use 3